PEDIATRICS, CHILD AND ADOLESCENT HEALTH

CHILDHOOD AND ADOLESCENCE

TRIBUTE TO EMANUEL CHIGIER, 1928-2017

PEDIATRICS, CHILD AND ADOLESCENT HEALTH

JOAV MERRICK - SERIES EDITOR

NATIONAL INSTITUTE OF CHILD HEALTH AND HUMAN DEVELOPMENT, MINISTRY OF SOCIAL AFFAIRS, JERUSALEM

Childhood and Adolescence: Tribute to Emanuel Chigier, 1928-2017
Joav Merrick (Editor)
2018. ISBN: 978-1-53613-574-9 (Hardcover)
2018. ISBN: 978-1-53613-574-9 (e-book)

Child Health and Human Development Yearbook 2017
Joav Merrick (Editor)
2018. ISBN: 978-1-53613-628-9 (Hardcover)
2018. ISBN: 978-1-53613-629-6 (e-book)

Child and Adolescent Health Yearbook 2017
Joav Merrick (Editor)
2018. ISBN: 978-1-53613-594-7 (Hardcover)
2018. ISBN: 978-1-53613-595-4 (e-book)

Chronic Disease and Disability: The Pediatric Gastrointestinal Tract
Donald E Greydanus, Orhan Atay, and Joav Merrick (Editors)
2018. ISBN: 978-1-53612-948-9 (Hardcover)
2018. ISBN: 978-1-53612-949-6 (e-book)

Multiple Sclerosis in Children and Adolescents
Hatim Omar and Joshua Chalkley (Editors)
2018. ISBN: 978-1-53612-979-3 (Hardcover)
2018. ISBN: 978-1-53612-980-9 (e-book)

Childhood and Adolescence: Tribute to Emanuel Chigier, 1928-2017
Joav Merrick (Editor)
2018. ISBN: 978-1-53613-574-9 (Softcover)
2018. ISBN: 978-1-53613-575-6 (e-book)

Chronic Disease and Disability: The Pediatric Lung
Donald E Greydanus, Myrtha M Gregoire-Bottex, Kevin W Cates and Joav Merrick (Editors)
2018. ISBN: 978-1-53613-577-0 (Hardcover)
2018. ISBN: 978-1-53613-578-7 (e-book)

Bicycles: Helmet Use of Adolescents at Independent Schools
Ronald Chow, Michael Borean, Drew Hollenberg, Jaclyn Viehweger, Tharani Anpalagan and Anna Rzepka (Editors)
2017. ISBN: 978-1-53612-458-3 (Hardcover)
2017. ISBN: 978-1-53612-459-0 (e-book)

Positive Youth Development: Long Term Effects in a Chinese Program
Daniel TL Shek, Cecilia MS Ma, Janet TY Leung and Joav Merrick (Editors)
2017. ISBN: 978-1-53612-539-9 (Hardcover)
2017. ISBN: 978-1-53612-540-5 (e-book)

Adolescence: Bicycle and Helmet Use of Adolescents and Young Adults
Ronald Chow and Joav Merrick (Editors)
2017. ISBN: 978-1-53612-039-4 (Hardcover)
2017. ISBN: 978-1-53612-060-8 (e-book)

Suicide: A Global View on Suicidal Ideation among Adolescents
Mazyanga L. Mazaba, Seter Siziya and Joav Merrick (Editors)
2017. ISBN: 978-1-53611-788-2 (Hardcover)
2017. ISBN: 978-1-53611-799-8 (e-book)

Children and Youth: Post-Traumatic Stress Disorder and Motor Vehicle Crashes
Donald E. Greydanus, Roger W. Apple, Kathryn White, and Joav Merrick (Editors)
2017. ISBN: 978-1-53611-102-6 (Hardcover)
2017. ISBN: 978-1-53611-255-9 (e-book)

Child and Adolescent Health Yearbook 2016
Joav Merrick (Editor)
2017. ISBN: 978-1-53610-948-1 (Hardcover)
2017. ISBN: 978-1-53610-957-3 (e-book)

Child Health and Human Development Yearbook 2016
Joav Merrick (Editor)
2017. ISBN: 978-1-53610-946-7 (Hardcover)
2017. ISBN: 978-1-53610-958-0 (e-book)

Chronic Disease and Disability: The Pediatric Kidney
Donald E Greydanus, Vimal Master Sankar Raj, and Joav Merrick (Editors)
2016. ISBN: 978-1-63483-793-4 (Hardcover)
2015. ISBN: 978-1-63483-809-2 (e-book)

Child and Adolescent Health Yearbook 2015
Joav Merrick (Editor)
2016. ISBN: 978-1-63484-512-0 (Hardcover)
2016. ISBN: 978-1-63484-543-4 (e-book)

Child Health and Human Development Yearbook 2015
Joav Merrick (Editor)
2016. ISBN: 978-1-63484-513-7 (Hardcover)
2016. ISBN: 978-1-63484-544-1 (e-book)

Pain Management Yearbook 2015
Joav Merrick (Editor)
2016. ISBN: 978-1-63484-515-1 (Hardcover)
2016. ISBN: 978-1-63484-545-8 (e-book)

Children and Childhood: Some International Aspects
Joav Merrick (Editor)
2016. ISBN: 978-1-63484-587-8 (Hardcover)
2016. ISBN: 978-1-63484-594-6 (e-book)

Children and Adolescents: Future Challenges
Daniel TL Shek, Tak Yan Lee, and Joav Merrick (Editors)
2016. ISBN: 978-1-63484-616-5 (Hardcover)
2016. ISBN: 978-1-63484-627-1 (e-book)

Adolescence: Positive Youth Development Programs in Chinese Communities
Daniel TL Shek, Florence KY Wu, Janet TY Leung, and Joav Merrick (Editors)
2016. ISBN: 978-1-63484-044-6 (Hardcover)
2016. ISBN: 978-1-63484-677-6 (e-book)

Sexuality: Some International Aspects
Joav Merrick and Donald E Greydanus (Editors)
2016. ISBN: 978-1-63484-707-0 (Hardcover)
2016. ISBN: 978-1-63484-719-3 (e-book)

Growing Up in the Middle East: The Daily Lives and Well-Being of Israeli and Palestinian Youth
Yossi Harel-Fisch, Ziad Abdeen and Miriam Navot
2016. ISBN: 978-1-63484-746-9 (Hardcover)
2016. ISBN: 978-1-63484-765-0 (e-book)

Chronic Disease and Disability: The Pediatric Heart
Donald E Greydanus, Devika Malhotra and Joav Merrick (Editors)
2016. ISBN: 978-1-63484-828-2 (Hardcover)
2016. ISBN: 978-1-63484-842-8 (e-book)

Diabetes Mellitus: Childhood and Adolescence
Manmohan K Kamboj, Donald E Greydanus and Joav Merrick (Editors)
2016. ISBN: 978-1-53610-095-2 (Hardcover)
2016. ISBN: 978-1-53610-104-1 (e-book)

Chronic Disease and Disability: Abuse and Neglect in Childhood and Adolescence
Donald E Greydanus, Vincent J Palusci and Joav Merrick (Editors)
2016. ISBN: 978-1-53610-129-4 (Hardcover)
2016. ISBN: 978-1-53610-142-3 (e-book)

Clinical Aspects of Psychopharmacology in Childhood and Adolescence, Second Edition
Donald E Greydanus, Joseph L Calles, Jr, Dilip R Patel, Ahsan Nazeer and Joav Merrick (Editors)
2016. ISBN: 978-1-53610-241-3 (Hardcover)
2016. ISBN: 978-1-53610-253-6 (e-book)

Chronic Disease and Disability: The Pediatric Pancreas
Donald E Greydanus, Manmohan K Kamboj and Joav Merrick (Editors)
2016. ISBN: 978-1-53610-055-6 (Hardcover)
2016. ISBN: 978-1-53610-065-5 (e-book)

A Pediatric Resident Pocket Guide: Making the Most of Morning Reports
Arthur N Feinberg
2015. ISBN: 978-1-63482-141-4 (Softcover)
2015. ISBN: 978-1-63482-186-5 (e-book)

Tropical Pediatrics: A Public Health Concern of International Proportions Second Edition
Richard R Roach, Donald E Greydanus, Dilip R Patel and Joav Merrick (Editors)
2015. ISBN: 978-1-63463-381-9 (Hardcover)
2015. ISBN: 978-1-63463-404-5 (e-book)

Child and Adolescent Health Issues (A Tribute to the Pediatrician Donald E Greydanus)
Joav Merrick (Editor)
2015. ISBN: 978-1-63463-574-5 (Hardcover)
2015. ISBN: 978-1-63463-576-9 (e-book)

Child and Adolescent Health Yearbook 2014
Joav Merrick (Editor)
2015. ISBN: 978-1-63482-162-9 (Hardcover)
2015. ISBN: 978-1-63482-206-0 (e-book)

Child Health and Human Development Yearbook 2014
Joav Merrick (Editor)
2015. ISBN: 978-1-63482-163-6 (Hardcover)
2015. ISBN: 978-1-63482-207-7 (e-book)

Behavioral Pediatrics, 4th Edition
Donald E Greydanus, Dilip R Patel, Helen D Pratt, Joseph L Calles Jr, Ahsan Nazeer and Joav Merrick (Editors)
2015. ISBN: 978-1-63483-027-0 (Hardcover)
2015. ISBN: 978-1-63483-052-2 (e-book)

Disability, Chronic Disease and Human Development
Joav Merrick
2015. ISBN: 978-1-63483-029-4 (Hardcover)
2015. ISBN: 978-1-63483-057-7 (e-book)

Caribbean Adolescents: Some Public Health Concerns
Cecilia Hegamin-Younge and Joav Merrick (Editors)
2015. ISBN: 978-1-63483-341-7 (Hardcover)
2015. ISBN: 978-1-63483-343-1 (e-book)

Adolescence and Health: Some International Perspectives
Joav Merrick (Editor)
2015. ISBN: 978-1-63483-791-0 (Hardcover)
2015. ISBN: 978-1-63483-808-5 (e-book)

Youth Suicide Prevention: Everybody's Business
Hatim A Omar (Editor)
2015. ISBN: 978-1-63483-786-6 (Softcover)
2015. ISBN: 978-1-63483-820-7 (e-book)

Human Developmental Research: Experience from Research in Hong Kong
Daniel TL Shek, Cecilia Ma, Yu Lu and Joav Merrick (Editors)
2014. ISBN: 978-1-62808-166-4 (Hardcover)
2013. ISBN: 978-1-62808-167-1 (e-book)

School, Adolescence and Health Issues
Joav Merrick, Ariel Tenenbaum and Hatim A Omar (Editors)
2014. ISBN: 978-1-62948-702-1 (Hardcover)
2014. ISBN: 978-1-62948-707-6 (e-book)

Adolescence and Sexuality: International Perspectives
Joav Merrick, Ariel Tenenbaum and Hatim A Omar (Editors)
2014. ISBN: 978-1-62948-711-3 (Hardcover)
2014. ISBN: 978-1-62948-724-3 (e-book)

Child and Adolescent Health Yearbook 2013
Joav Merrick (Editor)
2014. ISBN: 978-1-63117-658-6 (Hardcover)
2014. ISBN: 978-1-63117-668-5 (e-book)

Adoption: The Search for a New Parenthood
Gary Diamond and Eva Arbel (Israel)
2014. ISBN: 978-1-63117-710-1 (Hardcover)
2014. ISBN: 978-1-63117-713-2 (e-book)

Adolescence: Places and Spaces
Myra F Taylor, Julie Ann Pooley and Joav Merrick (Editors)
2014. ISBN: 978-1-63117-847-4 (Hardcover)
2014. ISBN: 978-1-63117-850-4 (e-book)

Pain Management Yearbook 2013
Joav Merrick (Editor)
2014. ISBN: 978-1-63117-944-0 (Hardcover)
2014. ISBN: 978-1-63117-959-4 (e-book)

Child Health and Human Development Yearbook 2013
Joav Merrick (Editor)
2014. ISBN: 978-1-63117-939-6 (Hardcover)
2013. ISBN: 978-1-63117-958-7 (e-book)

Born into this World: Health Issues
Donald E Greydanus, Arthur N Feinberg, and Joav Merrick (Editors)
2014. ISBN: 978-1-63321-667-9 (Hardcover)
2014. ISBN: 978-1-63321-669-3 (e-book)

Caring for the Newborn: A Comprehensive Guide for the Clinician
Donald E Greydanus, Arthur N Feinberg and Joav Merrick (Editors)
2014. ISBN: 978-1-63321-760-7 (Hardcover)
2014. ISBN: 978-1-63321-781-2 (e-book)

Environment and Hope: Improving Health, Reducing AIDS and Promoting Food Security in the World
Leslie Rubin and Joav Merrick (Editors)
2014. ISBN: 978-1-63321-772-0 (Hardcover)
2014. ISBN: 978-1-63321-782-9 (e-book)

Pediatric and Adolescent Dermatology: Some Current Issues
Donald E Greydanus, Arthur N Feinberg and Joav Merrick (Editors)
2014. ISBN: 978-1-63321-853-6 (Hardcover)
2014. ISBN: 978-1-63321-863-5 (e-book)

Adolescence and Behavior Issues in a Chinese Context
Daniel TL Shek, Rachel CF Sun, and Joav Merrick (Editors)
2013. ISBN: 978-1-62618-614-9 (Hardcover)
2013. ISBN: 978-1-62618-692-7 (e-book)

Advances in Preterm Infant Research
Jing Sun, Nicholas Buys and Joav Merrick
2013. ISBN: 978-1-62618-696-5 (Hardcover)
2013. ISBN: 978-1-62618-775-7 (e-book)

Child Health and Human Development: Social, Economic and Environmental Factors
Leslie Rubin and Joav Merrick (Editors)
2013. ISBN: 978-1-62948-166-1 (Hardcover)
2013. ISBN: 978-1-62948-169-2 (e-book)

Children, Violence and Bullying: International Perspectives
Joav Merrick, Isack Kandel and Hatim A Omar (Editors)
2013. ISBN: 978-1-62948-342-9 (Hardcover)
2013. ISBN: 978-1-62948-345-0 (e-book)

Chinese Adolescent Development: Economic Disadvantages, Parents and Intrapersonal Development
Daniel TL Shek, Rachel CF Sun and Joav Merrick (Editors)
2013. ISBN: 978-1-62618-622-4 (Hardcover)
2013. ISBN: 978-1-62618-694-1 (e-book)

Chronic Disease and Disability in Childhood
Joav Merrick
2013. ISBN: 978-1-62808-865-6 (Hardcover)
2013. ISBN: 978-1-62808-868-7 (e-book)

Environmental Health Disparities in Children: Asthma, Obesity and Food
Leslie Rubin and Joav Merrick (Editors)
2013. ISBN: 978-1-62948-122-7 (Hardcover)
2013. ISBN: 978-1-62948-135-7 (e-book)

Environmental Health: Home, School and Community
Leslie Rubin and Joav Merrick (Editors)
2013. ISBN: 978-1-62948-155-5 (Hardcover)
2013. ISBN: 978-1-62948-158-6 (e-book)

Guidelines for the Healthy Integration of the Ill Child in the Educational System: Experience from Israel
Yosefa Isenberg
2013. ISBN: 978-1-62808-350-7 (Hardcover)
2013. ISBN: 978-1-62808-353-8 (e-book)

Internet Addiction: A Public Health Concern in Adolescence
Artemis Tsitsika, Mari Janikian, Donald E Greydanus, Hatim A Omar and Joav Merrick (Editors)
2013. ISBN: 978-1-62618-925-6 (Hardcover)
2013. ISBN: 978-1-62618-959-1 (e-book)

Playing with Fire: Children, Adolescents and Firesetting
Hatim A. Omar, Carrie Howell Bowling and Joav Merrick (Editors)
2013. ISBN: 978-1-62948-471-6 (Softcover)
2013. ISBN: 978-1-62948-474-7 (e-book)

Promotion of Holistic Development of Young People in Hong Kong
Daniel TL Shek, Tak Yan Lee and Joav Merrick (Editors)
2013. ISBN: 978-1-62808-019-3 (Hardcover)
2013. ISBN: 978-1-62808-040-7 (e-book)

University and College Students: Health and Development Issues for the Leaders of Tomorrow
Daniel TL Shek, Rachel CF and Joav Merrick (Editors)
2013. ISBN: 978-1-62618-586-9 (Hardcover)
2013. ISBN: 978-1-62618-612-5 (e-book)

Break the Cycle of Environmental Health Disparities: Maternal and Child Health Aspects
Leslie Rubin and Joav Merrick (Editors)
2013. ISBN: 978-1-62948-107-4 (Hardcover)
2013. ISBN: 978-1-62948-133-3 (e-book)

Child and Adolescent Health Yearbook 2012
Joav Merrick (Editor)
2012. ISBN: 978-1-61942-788-4 (Hardcover)
2012. ISBN: 978-1-61942-789-1 (e-book)

Child Health and Human Development Yearbook 2011
Joav Merrick (Editor)
2012. ISBN: 978-1-61942-969-7 (Hardcover)
2012. ISBN: 978-1-61942-970-3 (e-book)

Child and Adolescent Health Yearbook 2011
Joav Merrick (Editor)
2012. ISBN: 978-1-61942-782-2 (Hardcover)
2012. ISBN: 978-1-61942-783-9 (e-book)

Tropical Pediatrics: A Public Health Concern of International Proportions
Richard R Roach, Donald E Greydanus, Dilip R Patel, Douglas N Homnick and Joav Merrick (Editors)
2012. ISBN: 978-1-61942-831-7 (Hardcover)
2012. ISBN: 978-1-61942-840-9 (e-book)

Child Health and Human Development Yearbook 2012
Joav Merrick (Editor)
2012. ISBN: 978-1-61942-978-9 (Hardcover)
2012. ISBN: 978-1-61942-979-6 (e-book)

Developmental Issues in Chinese Adolescents
Daniel TL Shek, Rachel CF Sun and Joav Merrick (Editors)
2012. ISBN: 978-1-62081-262-4 (Hardcover)
2012. ISBN: 978-1-62081-270-9 (e-book)

Positive Youth Development: Theory, Research and Application
Daniel TL Shek, Rachel CF Sun and Joav Merrick (Editors)
2012. ISBN: 978-1-62081-305-8 (Hardcover)
2012. ISBN: 978-1-62081-347-8 (e-book)

Understanding Autism Spectrum Disorder: Current Research Aspects
Ditza A Zachor and Joav Merrick (Editors)
2012. ISBN: 978-1-62081-353-9 (Hardcover)
2012. ISBN: 978-1-62081-390-4 (e-book)

Positive Youth Development: A New School Curriculum to Tackle Adolescent Developmental Issues
Hing Keung Ma, Daniel TL Shek and Joav Merrick (Editors)
2012. ISBN: 978-1-62081-384-3 (Hardcover)
2012. ISBN: 978-1-62081-385-0 (e-book)

Transition from Pediatric to Adult Medical Care
David Wood, John G Reiss, Maria E Ferris, Linda R Edwards and Joav Merrick (Editors)
2012. ISBN: 978-1-62081-409-3 (Hardcover)
2012. ISBN: 978-1-62081-412-3 (e-book)

PEDIATRICS, CHILD AND ADOLESCENT HEALTH

CHILDHOOD AND ADOLESCENCE

TRIBUTE TO EMANUEL CHIGIER, 1928-2017

JOAV MERRICK
EDITOR

nova
Medical & Health

Library of Congress Cataloging-in-Publication Data

ISBN: 978-1-53613-574-9
Library of Congress Control Number: 2018942245

Published by Nova Science Publishers, Inc. † New York

Contents

Introduction 1

Chapter 1 Emanuel Chigier, pediatrician, 1928-2017 3
Daniel Hardoff and Joav Merrick

Section one: Public health aspects 9

Chapter 2 The quest for an alternative paradigm of STEM education for young people 11
Daniel TL Shek and Po Chung

Chapter 3 Assessment and intervention for perinatal bonding disorder 33
Miki Mizumoto and Yoshiyuki Tachibana

Chapter 4 Measuring child survival in Trinidad: Preparation for Sustainable Development Goal 3 47
Kameel Mungrue, Katavia Balfour, Binta Baptiste, Asa Badall and Analiese Bates

Chapter 5 Training of potential program implementers for the Tin Ka Ping P.A.T.H.S. Project in China: Subjective outcome evaluation findings 65
Daniel TL Shek, Janet TY Leung, Lawrence K Ma, Li Lin and Florence KY Wu

Chapter 6 A qualitative study on the role of gender in the health and development of adolescents in disadvantaged communities in Ibadan, Nigeria **91**
Adesola O Olumide and Oladosu A Ojengbede

Chapter 7 Overparenting from the perspectives of Chinese parents and youths **115**
Janet TY Leung, Daniel TL Shek and Lorrie SL Ng

Chapter 8 Mothers' attributions in the relationship between young children's temperament and parenting stress **137**
Melissa Middleton and Kimberly Renk

Chapter 9 Does Head and Neck Cancer (HNC) Education Have an Impact on Adolescents' Knowledge and Attitude Towards HNC and HNC Peer Education? An Example from Nigeria **167**
Kehinde K Kanmodi and Omotayo F Fagbule

Chapter 10 Secondhand tobacco smoke exposure and attitudes towards the tobacco ban: A pilot survey of secondary school students in Ibokun Town, Nigeria **177**
Omotayo F Fagbule, Kehinde K Kanmodi and Timothy O Aladelusi

Chapter 11 Anaemia in infants: Is it always an 'iron clad' issue? An observational study **187**
Lutfi Jaber and Gary Diamond

Chapter 12 Child abuse and alcohol misuse in a victim: The role of ethnic and societal factors **205**
Sergei V Jargin

Chapter 13 Incidental oral hairy leucoplakia (OHL) in a healthy asymptomatic individual **215**
Lyubov Matytsina-Quinlan, Mrinalini Mahto, Donald E Greydanus and Laura Gwatkin

Section two: Acknowledgments **223**

Chapter 14 About the author **225**

Chapter 15 About the National Institute of Child Health and Human Development in Israel **227**

Chapter 16 About the book series "Pediatrics, child and adolescent health" **231**

Section five: Index **237**

Index **239**

INTRODUCTION

In: Childhood and Adolescence
Editor: Joav Merrick
ISBN: 978-1-53613-574-9

Chapter 1

EMANUEL CHIGIER, PEDIATRICIAN, 1928-2017

Daniel Hardoff[1,*], MD
and Joav Merrick[2-6], MD, MMedSci, DMSc
[1]Israel Center for Medical Simulation, Chaim Sheba Medical Center, Tel Hashomer, Israel
[2]National Institute of Child Health and Human Development, Jerusalem, Israel
[3]Health Services, Division for Intellectual and Developmental Disabilities, Ministry of Social Affairs and Social Services, Jerusalem, Israel
[4]Department of Pediatrics, Mt Scopus Campus, Hadassah Hebrew University Medical Center, Jerusalem, Israel
[5]Kentucky Children's Hospital, University of Kentucky, Lexington, Kentucky, US
[6]Center for Healthy Development, School of Public Health, Georgia State University, Atlanta, Georgia, US

---

[*]Correspondence: Daniel Hardoff, MD, 20 Lilach Street, IL-45203 HodHasharon, Israel. Email: drhardoff@gmail.com.

During a lifetime you meet many people and a few have a major impact on your own life and path that you will follow afterwards. We owe a lot of gratitude and debt to Manny (the Israeli pediatrician Emanuel Chigier, 1928-2017) for his inspiration, mentorship and friendship that will follow us for all our life and we give a big salute to Manny when he has now left us.

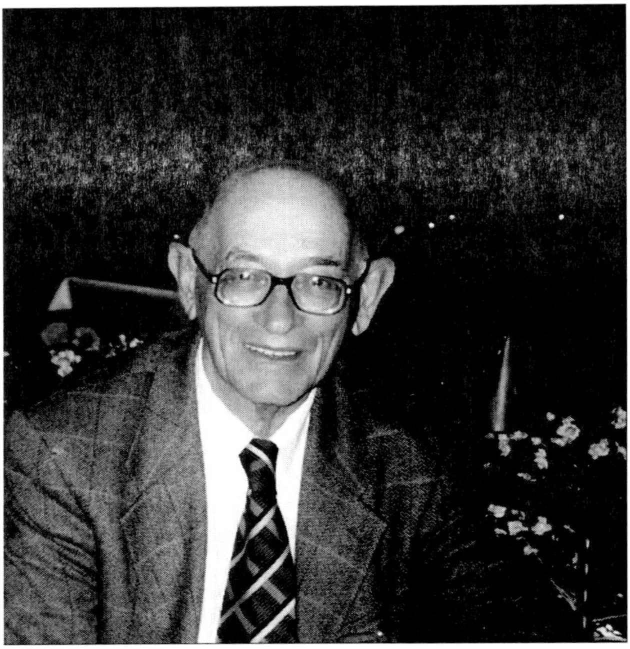

Emanuel Chigier.

INTRODUCTION

On October 2nd, 2017 the first Israeli adolescent medicine pediatrician, Emanuel Chigier, MD, passed away at the age of 89 years. Members of the Israel Society for Adolescent Medicine as well as many national and international colleagues have always appreciated Dr. Chigier as the propagator of adolescent comprehensive health services and the unique concept of adolescent medicine in Israel and around the world.

Emanuel Chigier's professional career of over 60 years was devoted to the well-being of children and young people. Following graduation from medical school in Johannesburg South Africa (University of Witwatersrand), Dr. Chigier trained in pediatrics in Israel and in England (1). After eight years of service as a senior pediatrician in Tel Hashomer and Hadassah Tel-Aviv hospitals, Dr. Chigier initiated the health promotion of adolescents in Israel.

During the 1960s he was the medical officer for the school health services of the Tel-Aviv Municipality and afterwards for 28 years he served as the director of the Medical Services of the Youth Aliyah of the Jewish Agency. Besides being a consulting pediatrician for these health services Dr. Chigier was also dedicated to developing learning curricula in adolescent health for educational staffs working with newly immigrated or socially disadvantaged teenagers. His greatest contribution in this respect was the establishment of health education programs for adolescents arriving from Ethiopia during the 1980s and the beginning of the 1990s. He was also the first to publish a comprehensive book in Hebrew on sex education for youth.

National and International Adolescent Health

Emanuel Chigier ignited the initiative to establish a multi-professional Israeli Association for Adolescent Health and further in 1985 founded the International Journal for Adolescent Medicine and Health and became its first editor (1985-1999). As a prominent contributor to the promotion of adolescent health beyond Israel, he was also one of the founders of the International Association for Adolescent Health (IAAH) and served as its treasurer for eight years. He was also one of the founders and an active member of the International Chapter of the Society for Adolescent Health and Medicine (SAHM).

Rehabilitation

He expanded his professional activities toward rehabilitation of young people with disabilities with special emphasis on sexual education and treatment. He was nominated lecturer in human sexuality at the Sackler School of Medicine of the Tel Aviv University and further on became an advisor to the International Study Group on Adolescent Sexuality of the World Health Organization and appointed to its Expert Advisory Panel on Rehabilitation.

Seminars, Conferences and Connection

Emanuel Chigier was the organizer and chairman of several international seminars and conferences that addressed adolescent health, health education, sexuality and disability as well as rehabilitation of children and young people. His brilliant lecturing ability made him a frequently invited speaker in conferences worldwide on adolescent health issues and the rehabilitation of young people.

On a personal level, the connection and work I (Daniel Hardoff) had with Manny, as we called him, encouraged me to specialize in adolescent medicine and in the many years of friendship with Manny, he will always remain my professional godfather. My (Joav Merrick) personal contact started in the end of the 1990s when we together with Henry Horwitz of the ISAS (International Seminars) did several international conferences together on Down syndrome and Adolescent violence in Jerusalem and Tel Aviv. Due to this collaboration Manny told me that he would retire from his position in Youth Aliyah and also as the editor of the International Journal of Adolescent Medicine and Health (IJAMH) published by Freund Publishing House in Tel Aviv and suggested I could take over as Editor in Chief. I had already for many years been involved with international collaborations as a Council Member of the International Society for Prevention of Child Abuse and Neglect (ISPCAN) and Chair of theirJournal Committee, but never been a journal editor. This was indeed a challenge and after a few years I managed to get IJAMH recognized and indexed in Index Medicus/PubMed and it opened a whole new world to me in scientific and academic publication. Today I am still the Editor in Chief of IJAMH, which has been recognized as the international journal in adolescent medicine with now 6 issues per year and published by De Gruyter in Berlin. This initial work has resulted in further connections around the world and today I am also the editor of another six international paper journals and 17 on-line peer-reviewed journals and managed to expand my international network and friendship.

Conclusion

We wanted to give credo to this larger than life ambassador and decided to gather papers from various parts of the world and topics that would have interested Manny and we are sure he would be proud with this tribute to all his life long achievements.

In the path of life you meet many people and a few have a major impact on your own life and path that you will follow afterwards. We owe a lot of gratitude and debt to Manny for his inspiration, mentorship and friendship that will follow us for all our life and we pay a big salute to Manny when he has now left us. We wish his wife, Miriam (Mixie), strength and health and many years more with good memories.

Reference

[1] Bennett DL, Merrick J. Tribute to Emanuel Chigier. Int J Adolesc Med Health 2001;13(1):2-3.

SECTION ONE: PUBLIC HEALTH ASPECTS

In: Childhood and Adolescence
Editor: Joav Merrick

ISBN: 978-1-53613-574-9

Chapter 2

THE QUEST FOR AN ALTERNATIVE PARADIGM OF STEM EDUCATION FOR YOUNG PEOPLE

Daniel TL Shek[1-6,*], PhD, FHKPS, BBS, SBS, JP and Po Chung[6], SBS, OBE, JP

[1]Department of Applied Social Sciences, The Hong Kong Polytechnic University, Hong Kong, PR China
[2]Centre for Innovative Programmes for Adolescents and Families, The Hong Kong Polytechnic University, Hong Kong, PR China
[3]Department of Social Work, East China Normal University, Shanghai, PR China
[4]Kiang Wu Nursing College of Macau, Macau, PR China
[5]Division of Adolescent Medicine, Department of Pediatrics, Kentucky Children's Hospital, University of Kentucky College of Medicine, Lexington, Kentucky, US

---

* Correspondence: Daniel TL Shek, PhD, FHKPS, BBS, SBS, JP, Associate Vice President (Undergraduate Programme), Chair Professor of Applied Social Sciences and Li and Fung Professor in Service Leadership Education, Department of Applied Social Sciences, The Hong Kong Polytechnic University, Hunghom, Hong Kong, PR China. Email: daniel.shek@polyu.edu.hk.

[6]Hong Kong Institute of Service Leadership and Management, Hong Kong, PR China

With the decline of competencies of science, technology, engineering and mathematics (STEM) in young people, there is a worldwide call for STEM education. While STEM education is important for young people, it is argued that it is equally important to nurture leadership attributes in young people based on an alternative version of STEM education. These STEM attributes include soft skills, trust, empathy and moral character. With the emergence of service economies, soft skills (particularly interpersonal cooperation and communication) and gaining trust from others are important attributes for adolescent development. With the decline in empathy in young people, there is a need to help young people understand the feelings and experience of other people. Finally, possessing good moral character is a core element of thriving youth development and successful leadership according to many theorists in different cultures.

INTRODUCTION

The acronym "STEM" stands for science, technology, engineering, and mathematics, which has received increasing attention on the agenda of educational reforms in the United States and many other countries in recent years. These four domains of STEM have been regarded as "cultural achievements that reflect people's humanity, power the economy, and constitute fundamental aspects of our lives as citizens, workers, consumers, and parents" (1). The term "STEM" was firstly used by the National Science Foundation in early 1990s and was subsequently used by numerous higher education institutions and academic communities.

The quest for STEM education has been propelled by two factors. First, the development of STEM education is largely driven by the challenge of globalization and global economic competition. As innovation-related industries have high potential to create more value-added jobs (2), STEM education is viewed by many countries as a strategy to address the needs to improve future employment prospects for the next-generation workers, which consequently increases national competitiveness (3). The second factor leading to the STEM movement is the widespread concern about the low STEM literacy amongst high school graduates in the United States (4). For example, according to the results of the Programme for International Student Assessment (PISA), American students only ranked in the middle in both math and science literacy out of 40 participating countries (5).

With specific reference to the decline in STEM literacy in the students in the United States, new initiatives have been proposed to foster the development of STEM education. Since the new millennium, several reports advocating STEM education have been published (6). In the report entitled "Rising Above the Gathering Storm" (7), the importance of designing a strong educational program to nurture innovative scientists and engineers in the 21st century is emphasized. In the "America COMPETES Act" in 2007, it is proposed to expand the existing STEM education programs and attention to technology and engineering (4,8). The Obama administration's "Race to the Top" competitive grant program clearly put STEM priority (9). In the initiatives entitled "A framework for K-12 Science Education" (10) and "Next Generation Science Standards" (11), significant provision of the integration of the four disciplines of STEM education is included.

While STEM education is as important as the development of scientific mindset and knowledge in young people, it alone does not help to nurture holistic development in young people. There are four reasons why STEM education alone is not enough. Primarily, from the holistic development perspective, skills and knowledge in the areas of science, technology, engineering and mathematics are just part of the education one should receive. Besides STEM, there are other areas of study, such as language, general education and physical education. Second, as there are research findings showing that positive development of young people, such as empathy and a sense of social responsibility, is declining, there is a need to re-think how we can promote positive development in young people. For example, there is research showing that empathy in young people is declining throughout the years while there has been an increase in egocentrism. Besides, Twenge and Donnelly (12) showed that there had been a shift in values from intrinsic motivation (e.g., learning for learning sake) to extrinsic motivation (learning for making money) from 1971 to 2014.

Third, it is obvious that the global economy is changing from an industrial mode to a post-industrial mode. In the industrial society, following orders (such as production in an assembly line) and top-down management are emphasized. On the other hand, workers are expected to be innovative and creative (i.e., not just following orders) and the supervisor-supervisee relationship is more egalitarian under the service economies (13). Against this background, one should ask what desired attributes young people should have under the service economies. For example, to have a smooth relationship between service providers and service recipients, one should have good communication skills. Besides, getting the trust from the service recipients and the co-workers is basic to transaction in service economies.

Finally, contemporary universities have been criticized for overlooking the traditional mission of universities. Twenge and Donnelly (12) explicitly remarked that colleges and universities are too market-driven. Dalton and Crosby (14) also pointed out that contemporary universities neglected the inner qualities of students, including value system, character, and social responsibility. Furthermore, employers have also criticized that contemporary university education fails to nurture graduates who can meet the demands of the real world.

In view of the above arguments, it is argued that besides STEM education in the science, technology, engineering and mathematics fields, we should look for an alternative version of STEM education for young people (soft skills, trust, empathy and moral character) which are important in the changing service economies. In terms of the requirements of service economies, these are essential attributes for leaders to provide quality service. From the perspective of positive youth development, these qualities are intrinsic to the optimal development of young people.

Soft skills

According to Rao (15), although the term "soft skills" was coined in the 1970s, it only gained renewed attention in the 1990s. As these skills are highly valued by employers, they are also regarded as "employability" skills. Generally speaking, while hard skills are formal, professional or technical knowledge which are commonly acquired through formal training, soft skills are informal, personal and implicit knowledge which may be acquired through formal and informal training. According to Grugulis and Vincent (16), soft skills include "communication, problem-solving, team-working, an ability to improve personal learning and performance, motivation, judgement, leadership and initiative" (16).

Besides, soft skills have been regarded as "transferable" skills which can be applied in different contexts. After synthesizing related materials in the literature, Andrews and Higson (17) suggested that transferable soft skills and competencies leading to employability include "ability to cope with uncertainty, ability to work under pressure, ability to plan and think strategically, capability to communicate and interact with others, either in teams or through networking, good written and verbal communication skills, information and communication technology skills, creativity and self-confidence, good self-management and time-management skills, and willingness to learn and accept responsibility" (17). According to the National Soft Skills Association, there are top ten soft skills as follows (http://www.nationalsoftskills.org/top-10-soft-skills-for-success):

- Dependability – degree of trust by others
- Motivation – energizing oneself to complete tasks and to motivate others and the organization
- Communication – skills that facilitate human interaction including both verbal and non-verbal communication skills
- Commitment – delivering the best and sense of loyalty to the tasks and the organization
- Creativity – seeing things and doing things from a new angle
- Problem Solving – handling issues and difficulties

Table 1. List of soft skills

1. Growth mindset	– readiness to improve oneself
2. Self-understanding	– strengths and weaknesses
3. Emotion regulation	– emotional management; emotional quotient
4. Self-confidence	– having faith in one's ability; self-efficiency
5. Stress management	– maintaining a balanced life during challenging situations; good emotional health
6. Resilience	– thrive under adversity; ability to bounce back in adversity
7. Ability to forgive and forget	– accept the mistakes of oneself and others; transcendence
8. Persistence and perseverance	– never give in or give up
9. Patience	– give time for things to take place
10. Perceptiveness	– be sensitive to people, environment, life and the tasks
11. Communication skills	– able to give and receive messages efficiently
12. Teamwork skills	– can work efficiently with different people
13. Interpersonal relationship skills	– social skills and interpersonal skills
14. Presentation skills	– effective presentation skills
15. Management skills	– effective ways to manage the organization
16. Facilitating skills	– integrate different views to form consensus
17. Selling skills	– facilitate buy-in
18. Team Building skills	– building an effective team
19. Leadership skills	– forming and passing on vision
20. Mentoring/coaching skills	– guide colleagues for career development
21. Managing upwards skills	– maintaining good relationships with one's supervisor
22. Self-promotion skills	– build up one's reputation
23. Skills in dealing with difficult personalities	– achieve outcomes although people are difficult
24. Skills in dealing with difficult/unexpected situations	– effective in view of difficulty
25. Savvy in handling office politics	– wisdom and skills in dealing with office dynamics
26. Influence/persuasion skills	– able to change others' views
27. Negotiation skills	– ability to get a "win-win" outcome
28. Networking skills	– ability to build up personal network

Note. 1-10 are self-management skills whereas 11-28 are people skills.

Han L. Soft skills list - 28 skills to working smart. Learn Soft Skills - Work Smart and Achieve More. Available at: https://bemycareercoach.com/soft-skills/list-soft-skills.html.

- Flexibility – open to different possibilities and easily adjusting to change
- Teamwork – ability to work together with others in a harmonious and efficient manner
- Leadership – guiding oneself, others and the organization
- Time Management – work-life balance, coping with workload and making priorities

According to Kechagias (18), there are 13 personal attributes and eight key skills in employability. For the personal attributes, they include loyalty, commitment, honesty and integrity, enthusiasm, reliability, personal presentation, common sense, positive self-esteem, sense of humor, balanced attitude to work and home life, ability to deal with pressure, motivation and adaptability. For the key skills, they include communication skills, team-work skills, problem-solving skills, planning and organizing skills and self-management skills. Other conceptual models on the contents of soft skills can be seen in Table 1 and Table 2.

Soft skills are also important from the perspective of potential employers. The 2013 Global Employability Survey (19) was conducted in 20 countries involving 2,700 respondents who were experienced managers. The objective was to understand their perceptions of the "ideal university" and "employable university graduate" from a corporate perspective. Regarding the top three attributes of an ideal university, they included "practical know-how," "integration of theories and practical knowledge," and "provision of soft skills." In fact, more than 90% of employers/managers maintained that an ideal university should include "soft skills" in its curriculum. Besides, personality, such as interpersonal skills and attitude, was regarded as the main success factor in a company and was more important than technical "know-how." According to the Times Higher Education (20), in a survey conducted by the Association of American Colleges and Universities, only one quarter of the employers felt that the graduates had good preparation in soft skills, such as critical thinking, logical reasoning, problem-solving and effective communication. Although soft skills were regarded as important attributes of university graduates, the students did not feel that the related education was adequate. The Higher Education Academy in the United Kingdom also conducted a student engagement survey amongst roughly 24,000 undergraduates (21). While the students reported that they had much gains in "hard skills," gains in "soft skills" (e.g., citizenship, creativity, and personal values) during their university years were little.

Table 2. 87 soft skills proposed by Mar (2016)

Communication Skills	**Influencing**	**Creativity**
1. Verbal Communication	31. Facilitation	61. Problem-solving
2. Body Language	32. Selling	62. Critical Thinking
3. Physical Communication	33. Inspiring	63. Innovation
4. Writing	34. Persuasion	64. Troubleshooting
5. Storytelling	35. Negotiation	65. Design Sense
6. Visual Communication	36. Motivating	66. Artistic Sense
7. Humor	37. Collaborating	
8. Quick-wittedness		
9. Listening	**Interpersonal Skills**	**Professional Skills**
10. Presentation Skills	38. Networking	67. Organization
11. Public Speaking	39. Interpersonal Relationships	68. Planning
12. Interviewing	40. Dealing with Difficult People	69. Scheduling
	41. Conflict Resolution	70. Time Management
Leadership	42. Personal Branding	71. Meeting Management
13. Team Building	43. Office Politics	72. Technology Savvy
14. Strategic Planning		73. Technology Trend Awareness
15. Coaching	**Personal Skills**	74. Business Trend Awareness
16. Mentoring	44. Emotional Intelligence	75. Research
17. Delegation	45. Self-awareness	76. Business Etiquette
18. Dispute Resolution	46. Emotion Management	77. Business Ethics
19. Diplomacy	47. Stress Management	78. Diversity Awareness
20. Giving Feedback	48. Tolerance of Change and Uncertainty	79. Disability Awareness
21. Managing Difficult Conversations	49. Taking Criticism	80. Intercultural Competence

Leadership	**Personal Skills**	**Professional Skills**
22. Decision Making	50. Self-confidence	81. Training
23. Performance Management	51. Adaptability	82. Train the Trainer
24. Supervising	52. Resilience	83. Process Improvement
25. Managing	53. Assertiveness	84. Knowledge Management
26. Manager Management	54. Competitiveness	85. Writing Reports and Proposals
27. Talent Management	55. Self-leadership	86. Customer Service
28. Managing Remote Teams	56. Self-assessment	87. Entrepreneurial Thinking
29. Managing Virtual Teams	57. Work-life Balance	
30. Crisis Management	58. Friendliness	
	59. Enthusiasm	
	60. Empathy	

Mar A. 87 soft skills (The big list). Simplicable 2016. Available at: http://training.simplicable.com/training/new/87-soft-skills.

Trust by others (dependability)

Interpersonal trust is very important in human social relationships. Without interpersonal trust, no in-depth social relationship can be formed. According to some theorists, interpersonal trust is a multidimensional concept. For example, Rotenberg (22) argued that trust includes reliability (i.e., the fulfillment of a promise), emotional response (i.e., reliance on others to refrain from engagement in inappropriate social behaviors), and honesty (i.e., telling the truth). Holmes and Rempel (23) maintained that trust in interpersonal relationship includes predictability (one's behavior is consistent), dependability (one is honest or reliable) and faith (one is responsive and caring intrinsically).

The quality of interpersonal relationship one encounters determines the nature of trust. For example, the experience of having a reliable caregiver affects children's expectations in social relationships and shapes children's future interactions with others (24). In adolescence, trust from other people is based on trust beliefs and trustworthy behaviors. Rotter (25) showed that individuals' trust beliefs were related to trustworthy behavior. If adolescents have low trust beliefs, they will engage in untrustworthy behaviors (e.g., not keeping promises and not respecting confidential information) which make them lose trust from others (26).

Trustworthiness is a virtue of adolescents and it is a psychosocial competence to be developed. Interpersonal trust is important for adolescent development for several reasons. First, through the development of interpersonal trust, young people would acquire an enhanced self-understanding such as their own trust beliefs and their trust behavior (e.g., keeping promises, being honest and reliable), and the process would help them develop their self-identity. Participants who had trust from peers also showed higher levels of prosocial behavior because such behavior is congruent with their attribute of trustworthiness (27).

Second, trust from others is vital to the formation and development of positive relationships with the significant-others, including parents, peers and teachers (28). There is evidence showing that interpersonal trust promotes positive peer relationship which leads to stronger social bonding (26). Rotenberg et al. (29) indicated that children who are trustworthy had more friends, were welcomed by others and had better peer relationships. Besides, Rotenberg and Boulton (26) showed that adolescents with high trustworthiness from peers were high in both trustworthiness and trust beliefs.

Third, trust by others can promote the psychological well-being of children and adolescents. Rotenberg et al. (29) found that interpersonal trust was negatively associated with depressive symptoms and loneliness but positively associated with self-esteem. In the academic domain, when a teacher trusts the students, the students tend to have good academic performance (30). Besides, trust between teachers and students mediated the relationship between school deprivation and academic achievement (31). Besides, lack of parental trust was associated with a higher risk of illegal and violent behavior in adolescents (32). In contrast, higher parental trust was related to lower engagement in sexual activity and lower risky sexual behavior (33).

Empathy

Empathy is an important developmental domain in human interaction. While some theorists regarded empathy as a one-dimensional construct (34), others argued that it is a multi-dimensional concept involving both emotional and cognitive components (35). Emotional empathy can be regarded as the ability to feel the emotions of others whereas cognitive empathy refers to the ability to understand others' thoughts (36). Davis (37) proposed "personal distress" as the third dimension which refers to having negative feelings when experiencing negative emotions of others.

Because of cognitive maturation in the adolescent years, young people begin to have better ability to perceive and understand others' emotions and thoughts (38), which contributes to empathy towards others. Besides, the changing social roles and escalation in social responsibilities help to promote the sensitivity of adolescents to others' thoughts and emotions. There are research findings showing that there was an increase in cognitive empathy amongst adolescents aged between 13 and 18 (39).

The development of empathy is important for several reasons. First, it helps to shape morality and social behavior among children and adolescents (40). Theoretically, researchers assume that empathy, especially affective empathy, is negatively associated with delinquent behaviors (41). Empirically, Jolliffe and Farrington (35) found that low emotional empathy was directly related to bullying amongst male adolescents (aged 13-17); aggressive adolescents also typically showed low levels of empathy (42). Research studies also show that high empathy inhibits aggression and anti-social behaviors in children and adolescents (43).

Second, empathy is positively associated with prosocial behaviors such as cooperation with others (44). According to Batson's empathy-altruism hypothesis (43), empathy strengthens altruism and the motivation to help which is supported by some studies (45). Research also shows that empathy has positive impacts on the adolescents through motivating prosocial behaviors, and prosocial behaviors in turn facilitate the adolescents to have better peer relationships (46), increased general well-being (47), and better school performance (48).

Third, empathy promotes positive development in adolescents. Research showed that empathy decreases anxiety and distress (49), and contributes to reduced violent behavior (50). Empathy also promotes adolescent development in the long run. In their 23-year longitudinal study, Allemand, Steiger and Fend (51) demonstrated that adolescent empathy at 12 to 16 years predicted social competencies at 35 years. Besides, research showed that empathy and emotional intelligence promote the emergence and effectiveness of leadership and entrepreneurship, with followers of empathic leaders experiencing less physical and psychosomatic symptoms (52).

Empathy is an important developmental ideal from the positive youth development (PYD) perspective (53). PYD is a strength-based approach that views youths as resources to be developed instead of problems to be solved. Roth and Brooks-Gunn (54) referred PYD to a "5 Cs" model which includes competence, connection, character, confidence, and caring. Among which, caring is defined as "a sense of sympathy and empathy for others" (54). Therefore, the development of empathy is indispensable for positive youth development. Hence, to nurture young people to be leaders, it is essential for them to develop their competence.

Moral character

In many cultures, children are taught to learn basic knowledge about survival. However, besides education for survival, many cultures also emphasize the importance of moral values regarding the differentiation between "good" and "bad." Generally speaking, educators, parents and the general public expect the children to possess the ability to differentiate between "right" and "wrong." Without such ability, the society will simply be chaotic without law and order. Hence, moral character is emphasized in many cultures.

Primarily, children and adolescents should acquire mature moral reasoning (i.e., ability to differentiate between right and wrong moral behavior). According to Kohlberg (55), there are three levels of moral development. In the pre-conventional level, moral behavior is driven primarily by physical consequences and considerations. In the first stage, human beings are driven by avoidance of punishment. For example, an adolescent does not cheat in examination because he/she does not want to be punished. In the second stage, human beings do good things because of rewards. For example, a student works hard in his/her studies because such good behavior would lead to desirable physical consequences such as scholarships. In the second level (conventional level), human moral behavior is governed by social norms and conventions. In the third stage, students perform good behavior because they will be praised by others. In other words, morality at this stage is "good boy or good girl" morality. In the fourth stage, a person does something good because of duty or obligation. For example, a student obeys the law because he/she knows that it is the duty of a citizen. According to Kohlberg, the moral development of many people stops at this stage (i.e., fulfilling the duties as a member of a community). As for the youth development, young people should be socialized to obey the law of the society and fulfill the basic duties of a citizen.

However, morality does not stop at the conventional level in Kohlberg's model. In the post-conventional level, a person acts in a moral manner because of reasons that transcend physical and social considerations. In Stage 5, a person's engagement in moral behavior is based on the "law behind the law" or the principle of social contract. For example, an adolescent does not spit not because of the fear of punishment or receiving bad comments from other people. Instead, he/she does not spit because he/she believes that this is not hygienic and may cause disease in the community. Hence, the law behind the law (i.e., social contract) is placed at the highest priority. In the final stage of Kohlberg's theory, it is proposed that a person will act in a moral manner according to the universal ethical principles, such as love and justice. For example, a person does not spit because he/she believes it is not an act of love. Obviously, the post-conventional level of moral development is developmental ideal for youth development. Young people should learn social contract as well as universal ethical moral principles.

Besides moral reasoning proposed by Lawrence Kohlberg, there are other views suggesting that young people should acquire moral competence. According to Catalano et al. (56), moral competence is a basic positive youth development construct which shapes the development of young people. It is defined as "a youth's ability to assess and respond to the ethical, affective, or social justice dimensions of a situation" and includes "a sense of right and wrong, or a sense of moral or social justice" (56). Similarly, Park and Peterson (57) argued that "moral competence among adolescents can be approached in terms of good character" (57). They further defined good character as "a family of positive traits reflected in thoughts, feelings and behavior" (57) and character strengths as the "subset of personality traits on which we place moral values" (58). Park, Peterson and Seligman (59) proposed that there are 24 universally-valued character strengths that can be subsumed under six dimensions. These include wisdom and knowledge (creativity, curiosity, love of learning, open mindedness, perspective), courage (authenticity, bravery, persistence, zest), humanity (kindness, love, social intelligence), justice (fairness, leadership, teamwork), temperance (forgiveness, modesty, prudence, self-regulation) and transcendence (appreciation of beauty and excellence, gratitude, hope, humor and religiousness).

Moral competence is also strongly emphasized in the leadership literature. According to Jormsri et al. (60), moral competence in nursing practice includes moral perception, moral judgment and moral behavior which has several dimensions including loving kindness, compassion, sympathetic joy, equanimity, responsibility, discipline, honesty, respect for human dignity, as well as values and rights. Similarly, Morales-Sanchez and Cabello-Medina (61) argued that there are four universal moral competencies which shape ethical decision-making. These competencies could be conceived as moral virtues which include prudence (e.g., reason, sagacity, docility, reflection and caution), justice (e.g., performance of fair acts, doing the "just" things), temperance (e.g., self-control, moderation, chastity, honesty, humility) and fortitude (e.g., patience, perseverance, moral courage). According to them, moral competence is character strength which is stable and can facilitate good behavior. Similarly, Gini and Green (62) argued that there are ten virtues of outstanding leaders, including deep honesty, moral courage, moral vision, compassion and care, fairness, intellectual excellence, creative thinking, aesthetic sensitivity, good timing, and deep selflessness.

Moral character is also strongly emphasized in the Chinese culture (63). In the Confucian thoughts, virtues are emphasized particularly in the development of children and adolescents. In "*ba de*" (eight cardinal virtues), the virtues include "*zhong*, *xiao*, *ren*, *ai*, *xin*, *yi*, *he*, *ping*" (loyalty, filial piety, benevolence, affection, trustworthiness, righteousness, harmony, peace). In "*si wei*" (four pillars of society), the virtues are "*li*, *yi*, *lian*, *chi*" (propriety, righteousness, integrity, shame). In "*wu chang*" (five constant virtues), the virtues include "*ren*, *yi*, *li*, *zhi*, *xin*" (benevolence, righteousness, propriety, wisdom, trustworthiness).

In particular, several virtues were emphasized in the traditional Chinese culture. First, strong emphasis is placed on the attainment of high morality. As stated in the *Great Learning*, "the way of great learning consists in manifesting one's bright virtue, consists in loving the people, consists in stopping in perfect goodness" (*daxue zhi dao, zai ming mingde, zai qinmin, zai zhiyu zhishan*). Similar emphasis can be seen in *Di Zi Gui* (64), "neither be harsh on myself, nor give up on myself; to be a person of high ideals, moral standards and virtue is something we can all attain in time" (*wu zibao, wu ziqi, sheng yu xian, ke xunzhi*).

Second, there was a strong emphasis on self-reflection, as exemplified in the Confucian principle of "*wu ri sanxing wushen*" (I daily examine myself on three points). In *Di Zi Gui*, it is maintained that "*jian ren e, ji neixing, you ze gai, wu jiajing. Wei dexue, wei caiyi, buru ren, dang zili*" (when I see others do wrong, I must immediately reflect upon myself. If I have made the same mistake, I will correct it. If not, I will take extra care not to make the same mistake. When my morals, conduct, knowledge, and skills seem not as good as those of others, I will encourage myself to be better).

Finally, there is a strong emphasis of trustworthiness ("*xin*") in the traditional Chinese culture. Basically, trust is fundamental to human interactions and is vital to intimate human relationships. As Confucius once said, "*ren er wu xin, bu zhi qi ke*" (I do not know how a man without truthfulness is to get on). Teaching children to have trustworthiness is also very important, as exemplified in *Di Zi Gui* - "*fan chuyan, xin wei xian, zha yu wang, xi ke yan*" (When I speak, honesty is important. Deceitful words and lies must not be tolerated).

While moral character is an important developmental outcome, there are several obstacles hindering its development in young people, particularly in Hong Kong. First, with the decline of the traditional Chinese cultural influence, moral development in young people is receiving less attention. Although some traditional values, such as filial piety, are still strong in Hong Kong, other traditional values, such as emphases on reflection and humility, have weakened. Second, as Hong Kong is a pragmatic society, materialism and academic achievement are strongly emphasized. In contrast, focus on spiritual values, such as putting the interest of others above oneself, is not the main trend. Third, with the emergence of post-modern thoughts, there is a view that morality is in fact socially constructed and there is no absolute right or wrong behavior because morality is basically relative. Fourth, with the rise of marital disruption and a fewer number of children in the family, family as an important base of moral socialization has weakened. Fifth, although moral education is included in the formal curriculum, it is not strongly emphasized because going to university does not depend on the moral behavior of a student. As a result, the importance of moral development in students is more a slogan than a well-implemented educational policy.

CONCLUSION

STEM education is important because these four elements are vital to the technological advance and human progress. STEM education aims to promote students' interests in these areas. For some theorists, they argue that STEM alone is not enough and they add "arts and design" in the acronym to make the whole thing as "STEAM." The basic argument is that STEM is without meaning without design concepts.

In this paper, it is proposed that an alternative form of STEM education is needed and the acronym stands for soft skills, trust, empathy and moral character. These attributes are important from two perspectives. First, from the holistic youth development perspective, the proposed elements are important for youth development. In fact, in many theories on positive youth development, the alternative STEM elements are emphasized. Second, with the changing global economy from manufacturing to service economies, the alternative STEM elements are important because of the intensive human interactions under service economies. Without soft skills (such as emotional quotient), trust, empathy and moral character, effective leadership in service economies would not be possible (13).

Acknowledgments

The authorship is equally shared between the two authors. The preparation for this paper is financially supported by the Victor and William Fung Foundation under the Li and Fung Endowed Professorship in Service Leadership Education. This is a re-published chapter based on an article published in the International Journal of Child and Adolescent Health.

References

[1] National Research Council. Successful K-12 STEM education: Identifying effective approaches in science, technology, engineering, and mathematics. Washington, DC: National Academies Press, 2011. URL: https://doi.org/10.17226/13158.

[2] Lacey TA, Wright B. Occupational employment projections to 2018. Mon Labor Rev 2009;132:82-123.

[3] Bybee RW. What is STEM Education? Science 2010;329(5995):996. URL: https://doi.org/10.1126/science.1194998.

[4] Sanders M. STEM, STEM Education, STEMmania. Tech Teacher 2009;68(4):20-7.

[5] OECD. Learning for tomorrow's world: First results from PISA 2003. 2004. URL: https://doi.org/10.1787/9789264006416-en.

[6] Kumtepe AT, Genc-Kumtepe E. STEM in early childhood education: We talk the talk, but do we walk the walk? In Information Resources Management Association, ed. STEM education: Concepts, methodologies, tools, and applications. Vol. 1. Hershey, PA: Information Science Reference 2015:1-24. URL: https://doi.org/10.4018/978-1-4666-7363-2.ch001.

[7] National Academies of Sciences. Rising above the gathering storm. Washington, DC: National Academies Press, 2005. URL: https://doi.org/10.17226/11463.

[8] Kuenzi JJ. Science, technology, engineering, and mathematics (STEM) education: Background, federal policy, and legislative action. Congress Res Serv 2008;35:1-31. URL: http://digitalcommons.unl.edu/crsdocs/35.

[9] Kolbe T, Rice JK. And they're off: Tracking federal race to the top investment from the starting gate. Educ Policy 2012;26(1):185-209. URL: https://doi.org/10.1177/0895904811428975.

[10] National Research Council. A framework for K-12 science education: Practices, crosscutting concepts, and core ideas. Washington, DC: National Academies Press, 2012. URL: https://doi.org/10.17226/13165.

[11] NGSS Lead States. Next generation science standards: For States, by States. Washington, DC: National Academies Press, 2013. URL: https://doi.org/10.17226/18290.

[12] Twenge JM, Donnelly K. Generational differences in American students' reasons for going to college, 1971–2014: The rise of extrinsic motives. J Soc Psychol 2016;156(6):620-9.

[13] Shek DTL, Chung PPY, Leung H. Manufacturing economy vs. service economy: Implications for service leadership. Int J Disabil Hum Dev 2015;14(3):205-15.

[14] Dalton J, Crosby P. Being and having: Shouldn't excellence in higher education (and people) be a measure of what one does rather than what one has? J Coll Character 2007;9:1-5.

[15] Rao MS. Enhancing employability in engineering and management students through soft skills. Ind Commerc Train 2014;46(1):42-8.

[16] Grugulis I, Vincent S. Whose skill is it anyway? 'soft' skills and polarization. Work Employ Soc 2009;23(4):597-615.

[17] Andrews J, Higson H. Graduate employability, 'soft skills' versus 'hard' business knowledge: A European study. High Educ Eur 2008;33(4):411-22.

[18] Kechagias K, editor. Teaching and assessing soft skills. 2011. URL: http://mass.educational- innovation.org/attachments/ 396_MASS%20wp4%20final %20report%20part-1.pdf.

[19] Emerging Associates, Trendence. Global Employability Survey and University Ranking 2013. 2013. URL: http://emerging.fr/Global%20employability%20survey %202013%20-%20Main%20report%20PDF.pdf.

[20] Times Higher Education. US universities should follow UK in promoting students' soft skills. 2015. URL: https://www.timeshighereducation.com/comment/opinion/us-universities-should-follow-uk-in-promoting-students-soft-skills/2019081.article.

[21] Buckley A. Students' perceptions of skills development. York: Higher Education Academy, 2015. URL: https://www.heacademy.ac.uk/sites/default/files/ukes_2015.pdf.

[22] Rotenberg KJ. Trust across the life-span. In Smelser NJ, Baltes PB, eds. International encyclopedia of the social and behavioural sciences. New York: Pergamon, 2001:7866-8.

[23] Holmes JG, Rempel JK. Trust in close relationships. In Hendrick C, ed. Review of personality and social psychology. Vol. 10. London: Sage, 1989:187-220.

[24] Bretherton I, Munholland KA. Internal working models in attachment relationships: A construct revisited. In Cassidy J, Shaver PR, eds. Handbook of attachment: Theory, research, and clinical applications. New York: Guilford, 1999:89-111.

[25] Rotter JB. Interpersonal trust, trustworthiness and gullibility. Am Psychol 1980;35:1-7.

[26] Rotenberg KJ, Boulton MJ. Interpersonal trust consistency and the quality of peer relationships during childhood. Soc Dev 2013;22(2):225-41.

[27] Malti T, Averdijk M, Zuffianò A, Ribeaud D, Betts LR, Rotenberg MJ, et al. Children's trust and the development of prosocial behavior. Int J Behav Dev 2016;40(3):262-70.

[28] Chin JC. Young children's trust beliefs in peers: Relations to social competence and interactive behaviors in a peer group. Early Educ Dev 2014;25(5):601-18.

[29] Rotenberg KJ, McDougall P, Boulton MJ, Vaillancourt T, Fox C, Hymel S. Cross-sectional and longitudinal relations among peer-reported trustworthiness, social relationships, and psychological adjustment in children and early adolescents from the United Kingdom and Canada. J Exp Child Psychol 2004;88(1):46-67.

[30] Goddard RD, Tschannen-Moran M, Hoy WK. A multilevel examination of the distribution and effects of teacher trust in students and parents in urban elementary schools. Elem Sch J 2001;102(1):3-17.

[31] Goddard RD, Salloum SJ, Berebitsky D. Trust as a mediator of the relationships between poverty, racial composition, and academic achievement. Educ Adm Q 2009;45(2):292-311.

[32] Melotti G, Potì S, Gianesini G, Brighi A. Adolescents at risk of delinquency. The role of parental control, trust, and disclosure. Deviant Behav 2017;1-16.

[33] Borawski EA, Ievers-Landis CE, Lovegreen LD, Trapl ES. Parental monitoring, negotiated unsupervised time, and parental trust: The role of perceived parenting practices in adolescent health risk behaviors. J Adolesc Health 2003;33(2):60-70.

[34] Eisenberg N, Strayer J. Critical issues in the study of empathy. In Eisenberg N, Strayer J, eds. Empathy and its development. New York: Cambridge University Press, 1987:3-13.

[35] Jolliffe D, Farrington DP. Is low empathy related to bullying after controlling for individual and social background variables? J Adolesc 2011;34:59-71.
[36] Gerdes KE, Segal E. Importance of empathy for social work practice: Integrating new science. Soc Work 2011;56:141-8.
[37] Davis MH. A multidimensional approach to individual differences in empathy. Catalog Select Doc Psychol 1980;10:85-103.
[38] Dumontheil I. Development of abstract thinking during childhood and adolescence: The role of rostrolateral prefrontal cortex. Dev Cogn Neurosci 2014;10:57-76.
[39] Blakemore S-J, Mills KL. Is adolescence a sensitive period for sociocultural processing? Annu Rev Psychol 2014;65:187-207.
[40] Hoffman ML. Empathy and moral development: Implications for caring and justice. New York: Cambridge University Press, 2000.
[41] de Wied M, Gispen-de Wied C, van Boxtel A. Empathy dysfunction in children and adolescents with disruptive behavior disorders. Eur J Pharmacol 2010;626:97-103.
[42] Lovett BJ, Sheffield RA. Affective empathy deficits in aggressive children and adolescents: A critical review. Clin Psychol Rev 2007;27:1-13.
[43] Batson CD, Ahmad NY, Stocks EL. Benefits and liabilities of empathy-induced altruism. In Miller AG, ed. The social psychology of good and evil. New York: Guilford, 2004:359-85.
[44] Ang RP, Goh DH. Cyberbullying among adolescents: The role of affective and cognitive empathy, and gender. Child Psychiatry Hum Dev 2010;41:387-97.
[45] Klimecki OM, Mayer SV, Jusyte A, Scheeff J, Schönenberg M. Empathy promotes altruistic behavior in economic interactions. Sci Rep 2016;6:31961. doi: http://dx.doi.org/10.1038/srep31961.
[46] Wentzel KR. Prosocial behavior and peer relations in adolescence. In Padilla-Walker LM, Carlo G, eds. Prosocial development: A multidimensional approach. Oxford: Oxford University Press, 2014:178-200.
[47] Weinstein N, Ryan RM. When helping helps: Autonomous motivation for prosocial behavior and its influence on well-being for the helper and recipient. J Pers Soc Psychol 2010;98(2):222-44.
[48] Caprara GV, Barbaranelli C, Pastorelli C, Bandura A, Zimbardo PG. Prosocial foundations of children's academic achievement. Psychol Sci 2000;11(4):302-6.
[49] Derksen F, Bensing J, Lagro-Janssen A. Effectiveness of empathy in general practice: A systematic review. Br J Gen Pract 2013;63:e76-84.
[50] Dodaj A, Sesar K, Barisic M, Pandza M. The effect of empathy on involving in bullying behavior. Cen Eur J Pediatr 2013;9:91-101.
[51] Allemand M, Steiger AE, Fend HA. Empathy development in adolescence predicts social competencies in adulthood. J Pers 2015;83(2):229-41.
[52] Humphrey RH. The benefits of emotional intelligence and empathy to entrepreneurship. Entrepre Res J 2013;3:287-94.
[53] Lerner RM, Almerigi JB, Theokas C, Lerner JV. Positive youth development: A view of the issues. J Early Adolesc 2005;25:10-6.

[54] Roth JL, Brooks-Gunn J. What is a youth development program? Identification and defining principles. In Jacobs F, Wertlieb D, Lerner RM, eds. Enhancing the life chances of youth and families: Public service systems and public policy perspectives. Handbook of applied developmental science: Promoting positive child, adolescent, and family development through research, policies, and programs. Vol. 2. Thousand Oaks, CA: Sage, 2003:197-223.

[55] Kohlberg L. Essays on moral development: The psychology of moral development. Vol. 2. San Francisco, CA: Harper Row, 1984.

[56] Catalano RF, Berglund ML, Ryan JA, Lonczak HS, Hawkins JD. Positive youth development in the United States: Research findings on evaluations of positive youth development programs. Prev Treat 2002;5:Article 15. doi:10.1037/1522-3736.5.1.515a.

[57] Park N, Peterson C. Moral competence and character strengths among adolescents: The development and validation of the Values in Action Inventory of Strengths for Youth. J Adolesc 2006;29:891-909. doi:10.1016/j.adolescence.2006.04.011.

[58] Park N, Peterson C. Positive psychology and character strengths: Application to strengths-based school counseling. Prof Sch Counsel 2008;12(2):85-92.

[59] Park N, Peterson C, Seligman MEP. Strengths of character and well-being. J Soc Clin Psychol 2004;23:603-19.

[60] Jormsri P, Kunaviktikul W, Ketefian S, Chaowalit A. Moral competence in nursing practice. Nurs Ethics 2005;12(6):582-94.

[61] Morales-Sanchez R, Cabello-Medina C. The role of four universal moral competencies in ethical decision-making. J Bus Ethics 2013;116:717-34.

[62] Gini A, Green RM. The ten virtues, in 10 virtues of outstanding leaders: Leadership and character. Oxford: Wiley-Blackwell, 2013. doi:10.1002/9781118551653.ch5.

[63] Shek DTL, Yu L, Fu X. Confucian virtues and Chinese adolescent development: A conceptual review. Int J Adolesc Med Health 2013;25(4):335-44. doi: 10.1515/ijamh-2013-0031.

[64] Pure Land Learning College Association. Di Zi Gui: Guide to a happy life. Toowoomba: Pure Land Books, 2005.

In: Childhood and Adolescence
Editor: Joav Merrick

ISBN: 978-1-53613-574-9

Chapter 3

ASSESSMENT AND INTERVENTION FOR PERINATAL BONDING DISORDER

***Miki Mizumoto**, PhD**
and Yoshiyuki Tachibana, MD, PhD
Division of Infant and Toddler Mental Health,
Department of Psychosocial Medicine, National Center
for Child Health and Development, Tokyo, Japan

Mothers with perinatal bonding disorder fail to form an emotional bond with their babies. This study outlines previous studies to shed light on the assessment of perinatal bonding disorder and appropriate intervention. We provide an overview of the symptoms that can lead to the suspicion of perinatal bonding disorder, tools for assessing bonding disorder, and the causes of bonding disorder. With regard to intervention for bonding disorder, indirect approaches targeting the psycho-social factors that affect maternal bonding (i.e., offering social support resources and enhancing maternal mental health and wellbeing) and direct approaches targeting the maternal bonding function (i.e., maternal sensitivity and the reflective function) are reviewed. As early intervention is suggested to be

* Correspondence: Miki Mizumoto, PhD, Department of Psychosocial Medicine, National Center for Child Health and Development, 2-10-1 Okura, Setagaya, Tokyo, 157-8535 Japan. Email: mkmizmo@yahoo.co.jp.

effective, there is a need for an assessment system that starts in the antenatal period. In addition, a comprehensive intervention system should be developed that allow all organizations to provide the necessary support for healthy mother-infant relationships.

INTRODUCTION

It is common knowledge that secure attachment is important for a child's healthy development. Attachment refers to a biological instinct in which proximity to an attachment figure is sought when the child senses or perceives threat or discomfort (1). Thus, "reactive attachment disorder" is a disorder that only exists in children and not in parents. For their healthy emotional growth, children must have secure attachment to a primary caregiver (in many cases, the mother). Thus, a maternal emotional bond, reflected by such statements as, "I love my baby," "She(he) is my own baby," and "I want to guard my baby from any risks," is indispensable. The development of this type of emotional bond is called "bonding"; for mothers, bonding also functions as a base for their continued involvement in child-rearing.

"Bonding disorder" describes a condition in which a mother fails to develop an emotional bond and rear their baby; this is different from "attachment disorder" (2). Although there is currently no distinct diagnostic category in the field of psychiatry, bonding disorder may lead to developmental deficiency in the child and to child abuse. Especially in the perinatal period, bonding disorder is a critical problem and represents a matter of life or death for the baby. Thus, it is important to assess bonding disorder and implement appropriate prophylactic intervention and treatment in the perinatal period. However, to date, few studies have comprehensively described the assessment of bonding disorder and appropriate intervention. The present study sheds light on the assessment of bonding disorder and appropriate intervention in the perinatal period by outlining previous studies.

THE ASSESSMENT OF BONDING DISORDER

Kumar noted (3) that the following emotions and behaviors are symptoms of bonding disorder: "alienation, indifference, detachment, and lack of love," and "resentment, hate and hostility" (3). Brockington (2) developed a postpartum bonding instrument and defined bonding disorder as "impaired bonding," "rejection and anger" and "anxiety about care" (2). These kinds of symptoms can be observed in both the prenatal and antenatal periods (4).

Despite the fact that bonding disorder is not included as a diagnosis in DSM-V or ICD-10, "relational disorder" (Diagnostic Classification: 0-3) (5), is similar to bonding disorder. In DC: 0-3, patients whose child rearing is considered "over-involved," "under-involved," "anxious/tense," or "angry/hostile" rearing may be diagnosed with "relationship disorder," even though they are not abusive.

The NICE (National Institute for Health and Care Excellence, United Kingdom) guidelines suggest that mothers with mental problems may experience difficulties with the mother-baby relationship, and recommends the assessment of "mother-baby relationships," such as verbal interaction, emotional sensibility, and physical care be included in the assessment of postnatal contact (6). However, bonding disorder can develop during pregnancy or in patients without current mental disorders. Moreover, because of the norm of maternal instinct, bonding disorder is difficult to detect. Thus, careful observations and interviews should be conducted by caregivers from the antenatal period to the postnatal period. Attention should be paid to the following symptoms:

- Indifference to the baby (fetus): In the antenatal period, the mother does not care about herself being pregnant. In the postnatal period, the mother does not hold the baby, does not breastfeed her baby or shows a lack of response to the baby even when he(she) cries. She seems to lack the maternal instinct.
- Rejection of the baby (fetus): During pregnancy, she appears to regret the pregnancy and acts as if she does not want to admit that

the pregnancy and delivery are a real matter. After delivery, the mother might say, "I do not think my baby is lovely," or "I do not think that I can raise my baby," and rejects caring for her baby.

- Anger at baby (fetus): The pregnant mother hits the stomach directing anger toward the fetus. After delivery, the mother is irritated that her baby does not stop crying or that her baby does not breastfeed, and shouts or curses at her baby.

Table 1. Tools for assessing bonding disorder

Methods	Tools	Description
Observation	Emotional Availability Scales (EAS) (7)	Observation of mother-child play. Parental dimensions: sensitivity, structuring, nonintrusiveness, nonhostility (cf. Child dimensions: responsiveness to parent, involvement of parent).
Interview to mothers	Working Model of the Child Interview (WMIC) (8)(9)	Semi-structured interview Interview mother to determine cognition of subjective experience in relation to baby and mother-infant relationships, and assess the parental representations.
	Birmingham Interview for Maternal Mental Health (10)	Semi-structured interview. Child's nature and maternal emotional availability are assessed.
Questionnaire to investigate maternal affection toward baby	The Postpartum Bonding Instrument (2)	6-point Likert scale, 25 items Subscales: impaired bonding, rejection and anger, anxiety about care, and risk of abuse.
	Mother-infant bonding questionnaire (MIBQ) (11)	4-point Likert scale, 10 items Subscales: loving, resentful, neutral or felt nothing, possessive, joyful, dislike, protective, disappointed, and aggressive.
	Postpartum maternal attachment scale (12)	4-point Likert scale, 21 items Subscales: core maternal attachment, anxiety regarding children.
	Mother-to-Infant Bonding Scale (MIBS) (13)	4-point Likert scale, 8 items A revised and simpler version of MIBQ (11)

Tools for Assessing Bonding Disorder

Tools for assessing bonding disorder are useful for identifying cases of bonding disorder, which is difficult to diagnose because mothers tend to hesitate to express their lack of an emotional bond with their babies (see Table 1 above).

Causes of Bonding Disorder

In order for appropriate intervention to be implemented in cases of bonding disorder, the cause of the disorder has to be assessed. The possible causes of bonding disorders can be categorized into three factors:

- Ecological factors: Separation from the baby, mother-child deprivation, lack of support, low social economic status, painful labor, unmarried mother, marital problems reported by mother, domestic violence.
- Maternal factors: Antenatal or postnatal depression, unwanted pregnancy, health problems in pregnancy, obstetric interventions (i.e., caesarean section, forceps delivery), painful labor, fearfulness, obsessive compulsiveness, immature personality, history of damaged early childhood, experience of stillbirth.
- Factors associated with the baby: Preterm, disease, disability, disappointment with the baby's gender, baby's nature (i.e., exploder or low reaction).

Intervention for Bonding Disorder

The NICE guidelines suggest that caregivers should discuss any concerns about the mother-baby relationship with the mother in whom bonding disorder is suspected, information should be provided for the mental health problem and treatment should be administered. If the problems in the relationship are not resolved, further intervention to improve the mother-baby relationship should be considered (6). Interventions should be based on the above-described causes of bonding disorder (1-3). Intervention for bonding disorder can be categorized into indirect and direct approaches (6, 14-16).

Indirect approach: Intervention targeting the psycho-social factors that affect maternal bonding

Offering social support resources like home visits by midwives, who provide information about pregnancy and child-rearing, and support by postpartum care center and helpers are included in this category (17-19). Caregivers themselves are supposed to be sources of support. Thus, relationships, which can be regarded as a "security base (an emotional base is important for mothers to develop healthy bonding with their babies)" from the perspective of attachment theory. Evidence of this kind of approach is only shown in relation to preventive intervention. If the mother has postpartum bonding disorder, it may difficult for her to be led to regional mental healthcare due to her relational problems. Thus, various efforts are needed in treatment measures that offer social support resources.

Evidence of secure attachment was reported in a study investigating the effects of home visits by volunteer coaches to low-income class primiparas (N=46) during pregnancy and for the first year after delivery in comparison to control group ($p<.001$) (17).

The Creating Opportunities for Parent Empowerment Program, which provides information about the appearance and behavioral characteristics of preterm infants and how to best parent them, was found to have significant effects on positive interactions between parents and their infants ($p<.05$, $d=.26$). In addition, parents showed stronger beliefs about their parental role ($p<.01$, $d=.36$), and about what behaviors and characteristics to expect from their children ($p<.001$, $d=.26$) (18).

Approaches to enhance maternal mental health and wellbeing are needed. Because bonding disorder might develop due to depression, it is effective to improve maternal mental health. This approach focuses on recovery from maternal mental disorders such as depression and fearfulness through psychotherapy. There is evidence of the effects of constructed psychotherapy (i.e., cognitive behavioral therapy, relational therapy and mindfulness programs).

A mindfulness program that included eight sessions for breastfeeding mothers and three sessions of psycho-education based on interpersonal psychotherapy (IPT) was found to enhance maternal self-efficacy (p<0.01) (20-22).

Non-directive counseling, cognitive behavioral therapy and psychodynamic psychotherapy have been offered; all such therapies led to the improvement of the mother-infant relationship at 4.5 months after birth (p<0.05) (23, 24).

The direct approach: Intervention targeting the maternal bonding function

A direct approach targeting the maternal bonding function is an approach that is unique to bonding disorder. A systematic review about interventions for first-year mothers targeting only maternal sensitivity or both sensitivity and the reflective function showed that the odds ratio of secure-type attachment was higher in cases in which both types of intervention were implemented in comparison to cases with no intervention or in which usual interventions were implemented (*OR*:2.77). However, the differences in the effects between approaches targeting only maternal sensitivity and those targeting both sensitivity and the reflective function were unclear (16).

Intervention targeting maternal sensitivity

Sensitive and responsive caregiving is the most powerful predictor of secure maternal-child attachment (25). Home visit using video-feedback intervention to promote positive parenting (VIPP) enhanced maternal sensitivity ($p<.05$, $d=.78$) (26), and improved the quality of the mother-infant relationships (27). Mother-infant relationship guidance that aimed to enhance sensitive and responsive mother-infant interaction was shown to improve maternal sensitivity and responsiveness, and the infant's attachment (28, 29).

Intervention targeting maternal sensitivity and the reflective function

The reflective function is the mother's ability to reflect on her own and her child's behavior, thoughts, and feelings in attachment/caregiving interactions, on her personal experience, and on the history affecting her current caregiving interactions. It is known that the reflective function is improved by focusing on maternal representations of attachment relationships with the mother's own parents and how those affect the present maternal representations of their children (30, 31). There is evidence to support the efficacy of intervention targeting maternal sensitivity and the reflective function in mothers who are considered to be at high risk due to factors such as low income, incarceration or abuse.

The perinatal version of a program called "Circle of security" (a program based on attachment theory that aims to encourage mothers to rear children securely) targeted pregnant mothers, who were in jail because of drug abuse ($N=20$). It was found to be effective for improving both maternal sensitivity and the child's attachment (child attachment was comparable to a normal population) (32). Circle of security HV4 (home visit version) was found to have an effect with regard to securing the attachment between mothers and hot-tempered children ($p<.05$) (33).

Project STEEP (Steps Toward Effective and Enjoyable Parenting) aimed to encourage maternal sensitivity, promote discussion on maternal attachment representation, and to enhance family support. STEEP provided evidence of more secure attachment in first-year infants (OR:3.1, $p=.002$), lower infant rearing risk for mothers of 24-month-old infants ($p=.002$), and reduced the incidence of disorganized attachment (34).

Mother-infant psychoanalytic psychotherapy for mothers with mental health problems and social hatred and their infants (younger than one year old) showed no effect in the period immediately after intervention; however, the intervention group showed less maternal infant rearing stress ($p=0.08$), better maternal representation ($p=0.05$), and better mother-infant relationships ($p=.031$) (35). VIPP-R, which was discussion on the association between current infant-rearing and the maternal attachment experience in the infant stage revealed that VIPP-R improved maternal sensitivity as well as VIPP (36-38).

In a systematic review on the abovementioned direct interventions, early intervention for bonding disorder affected maternal sensitivity ($d=.33$, $p<.001$), and the child's attachment ($d=.19$, $p<.05$) (sample: children <54 months of age, $N=9{,}139$, 70 studies). The most effective interventions were those that started when the infant was >6 months of age, programs that involved <16 sessions, and interventions that focused on sensitivity alone (39). On the other hand, a meta-analysis that studied the effects of interventions aimed at promoting maternal sensitivity and the maternal reflective function during the first year of the infant's life revealed that both types of intervention increased the odds of secure maternal-child attachment in comparison to no intervention or standard intervention ($N=1{,}678$, seven trials; odds ratio: 2.77). In particular, parent-infant psychotherapy for abusive parents and infants (40) showed the greatest effect (odds ratio: 40.18) (16).

CONCLUSION

We have reviewed the literature on assessment of bonding disorder and appropriate interventions, which is especially necessary in the perinatal period for producing secure attachment in the infants, and avoiding infantile abuse. Bonding disorder may be difficult to identify because of strong norm that maternal love exists due to instinct. It is important to recognize that mother-baby relational problems might exist in association with or separately from maternal mental health problems. A precise assessment that includes an assessment of the cause of the bonding disorder is necessary when deciding the approach with regard to mothers.

As early intervention is suggested to be effective, an assessment system that starts in the antenatal period should be developed. In addition, there is a need for a comprehensive intervention system that allows all organizations to provide necessary support for healthy mother-infant relationships.

Acknowledgments

This study was supported by Grant-in-Aid for Scientific Research from the Ministry of Health, Labour, and Welfare of Japan (H29-Sukoyaka-Ippan-004), and the Ministry of Education, Culture, Sports, Science, and Technology (Kiban C 15K09880).

References

[1] Bowlby J. Attachment and loss: Attachment. New York: Basic Books, 1969.

[2] Brockington I, Oates J, George S, Turner D, Vostanis P, Sullivan M, et al. A screening questionnaire for mother-infant bonding disorders. Arch Womens Ment Health 2001;3(4):133-40.

[3] Kumar R. Anybody's child: Severe disorders of mother-to-infant bonding. Br J Psychiatry 1997;171(2):175-81.

[4] Edhborg M, Nasreen H-E, Kabir ZN. Impact of postpartum depressive and anxiety symptoms on mothers' emotional tie to their infants 2–3 months postpartum: a population-based study from rural Bangladesh. Arch Womens Ment Health 2011;14(4):307.

[5] National Center for Clinical Infant Programs. Zero to three. Diagnostic classification 0–3. Diagnostic classification of mental health and developmental disorders of infancy and early childhood. Arlington, VA: NCCIP, 1994.

[6] NCCMH. Antenatal and postnatal mental health: The NICE guideline on clinical management and service guidance, Updated edition London: British Psychological Society, Royal College Psychiatrists, 2014.

[7] Biringen Z. Emotional availability: conceptualization and research findings. Am J Orthopsychiatry 2000;70(1):104.

[8] Zeanah CH, Barton ML. Introduction: Internal representations and parent-infant relationships. Infant Ment Health 1989;10(3):135-41.

[9] Zeanah CH, Benoit D, Barton M. Working model of the child interview. Unpublished manuscript, Brown University, RI. 1995.

[10] Brockington I, Guedeney A. Motherhood and mental health. London: Taylor Francis, 1999.

[11] Kumar R, Hipwell A. Development of a clinical rating scale to assess mother-infant interaction in a psychiatric mother and baby unit. Br J Psychiatry 1996;169(1):18-26.

[12] Nagata M, Nagai S, Sobajima H, Ando T, Nishide Y, Honjo S. Maternity blues and attachment to children in mothers of full-term normal infants. Acta Psychiatr Scand 2000;101(3):209-17.

[13] Taylor A, Atkins R, Kumar R, Adams D, Glover V. A new Mother-to-Infant Bonding Scale: links with early maternal mood. Arch Womens Ment Health 2005;8(1):45-51.

[14] Berlin LJ. Interventions to enhance early attachments: The state of the field today. In: Berlin LJ, Ziv Y, Amaya-Jackson L, Greenberg MT, eds. Duke series in child development and public policy. Enhancing early attachments: Theory, research, intervention, and policy. New York: Guilford, 2005:3-33.

[15] Egeland B, Weinfield NS, Bosquet M, Cheng V. Remembering, repeating, and working through: Lessons from attachment-based interventions. In: Osofsky JD, Fitzgerald HE, eds. WAIMH handbook of infant mental health. New York: 2000:35-89.

[16] Letourneau N, Tryphonopoulos P, Giesbrecht G, Dennis CL, Bhogal S, Watson B. Narrative and meta-analytic review of interventions aiming to improve maternal-child attachment security. Infant Ment health 2015;36(4):366-87.

[17] Jacobson SW, Frye KF. Effect of maternal social support on attachment: Experimental evidence. Child Dev 1991;62(3):572-82.

[18] Melnyk BM, Feinstein NF, Alpert-Gillis L, Fairbanks E, Crean HF, Sinkin RA, et al. Reducing premature infants' length of stay and improving parents' mental health outcomes with the Creating Opportunities for Parent Empowerment (COPE) neonatal intensive care unit program: a randomized, controlled trial. Pediatrics 2006;118(5):e1414-27.

[19] Morrell CJ, Slade P, Warner R, Paley G, Dixon S, Walters SJ, et al. Clinical effectiveness of health visitor training in psychologically informed approaches for depression in postnatal women: pragmatic cluster randomised trial in primary care. BMJ 2009;338: a3045.

[20] Perez-Blasco J, Viguer P, Rodrigo MF. Effects of a mindfulness-based intervention on psychological distress, well-being, and maternal self-efficacy in breast-feeding mothers: results of a pilot study. Arch Womens Ment Health 2013;16(3):227-36.

[21] Gao L-l, Chan SW-c, Li X, Chen S, Hao Y. Evaluation of an interpersonal-psychotherapy-oriented childbirth education programme for Chinese first-time childbearing women: A randomised controlled trial. Int J Nurs Stud 2010;47(10):1208-16.

[22] Gao L, Chan SW, Sun K. Effects of an interpersonal-psychotherapy-oriented childbirth education programme for Chinese first-time childbearing women at 3-month follow up: Randomised controlled trial. Int J Nurs Stud 2012;49(3):274-81.

[23] Cooper PJ, Murray L, Wilson A, Romaniuk H. Controlled trial of the short-and long-term effect of psychological treatment of post-partum depression. Br J Psychiatry 2003;182(5):412-9.

[24] Murray L, Cooper PJ, Wilson A, Romaniuk H. Controlled trial of the short-and long-term effect of psychological treatment of post-partum depression. Br J Psychiatry 2003;182(5):420-7.

[25] Ainsworth MDS, Blehar MC, Waters E, Wall SN. Patterns of attachment: A psychological study of the strange situation. New York: Psychology Press Routledge, 2015.

[26] Kalinauskiene L, Cekuoliene D, Van IJzendoorn M, Bakermans-Kranenburg MJ, Juffer F, Kusakovskaja I. Supporting insensitive mothers: the Vilnius randomized control trial of video-feedback intervention to promote maternal sensitivity and infant attachment security. Child Care Health Dev 2009;35(5):613-23.

[27] Van Doesum K, Riksen-Walraven JM, Hosman CM, Hoefnagels C. A randomized controlled trial of a home-visiting intervention aimed at preventing relationship problems in depressed mothers and their infants. Child Dev 2008;79(3):547-61.

[28] Barlow J, Davis H, McIntosh E, Jarrett P, Mockford C, Stewart-Brown S. Role of home visiting in improving parenting and health in families at risk of abuse and neglect: results of a multicentre randomised controlled trial and economic evaluation. Arch Dis Child 2007;92(3):229-33.

[29] Cooper PJ, Tomlinson M, Swartz L, Landman M, Molteno C, Stein A, et al. Improving quality of mother-infant relationship and infant attachment in socioeconomically deprived community in South Africa: randomised controlled trial. BMJ 2009;338: b974.

[30] Fonagy P, Steele M, Steele H, Moran GS, Higgitt AC. The capacity for understanding mental states: The reflective self in parent and child and its significance for security of attachment. Infant Ment Health 1991;12(3):201-18.

[31] Slade A, Grienenberger J, Bernbach E, Levy D, Locker A. Maternal reflective functioning, attachment, and the transmission gap: A preliminary study. Attach Hum Dev 2005;7(3):283-98.

[32] Cassidy J, Ziv Y, Stupica B, Sherman LJ, Butler H, Karfgin A, et al. Enhancing attachment security in the infants of women in a jail-diversion program. Attach Hum Dev 2010;12(4):333-53.

[33] Cassidy J, Woodhouse SS, Sherman LJ, Stupica B, Lejuez C. Enhancing infant attachment security: An examination of treatment efficacy and differential susceptibility. Dev Psychopathol 2011;23(1):131-48.

[34] Suess G, Bohlen U, Carlson E, Spangler G, Frumentia Maier M. Effectiveness of attachment based STEEP™ intervention in a German high-risk sample. Attach Hum Dev 2016;18(5):443-60.

[35] Fonagy P, Sleed M, Baradon T. Randomized controlled trial of parent–infant psychotherapy for parents with mental health problems and young infants. Infant Mental Health journal. 2016;37(2):97-114.

[36] Bakermans-Kranenburg MJ, Juffer F, Van Ijzendoorn MH. Interventions with video feedback and attachment discussions: Does type of maternal insecurity make a difference? Infant Ment Health 1998;19(2):202-19.

[37] Svanberg P, Mennet L, Spieker S. Promoting a secure attachment: A primary prevention practice model. Clin Child Psychol Psychiatry 2010;15(3):363-78.

[38] Klein Velderman M, Bakermans-Kranenburg MJ, Juffer F, Van Ijzendoorn MH. Effects of attachment-based interventions on maternal sensitivity and infant attachment: Differential susceptibility of highly reactive infants. J Fam Psychol 2006;20(2):266.

[39] Bakermans-Kranenburg MJ, Van Ijzendoorn MH, Juffer F. Less is more: meta-analyses of sensitivity and attachment interventions in early childhood. Psychol Bull 2003;129(2):195.

[40] Cicchetti D, Rogosch FA, Toth SL. Fostering secure attachment in infants in maltreating families through preventive interventions. Dev Psychopathol 2006;18(3):623-49.

In: Childhood and Adolescence
Editor: Joav Merrick
ISBN: 978-1-53613-574-9

Chapter 4

MEASURING CHILD SURVIVAL IN TRINIDAD: PREPARATION FOR SUSTAINABLE DEVELOPMENT GOAL 3

Kameel Mungrue**, MBBS, MPH, FRIPH, MBA, Katavia Balfour, MBBS, Binta Baptiste, MBBS, Asa Badall, MBBS and Analiese Bates, MBBS

Department of Paraclinical Sciences,
Public Health and Primary Care Unit, Faculty of Medical Sciences,
University of the West Indies, Mt Hope, Trinidad

Mortality in the age group under five years is an important health indicator, used as a measure of progress of human development around the world. This is because accurate statistics on infant mortality rates reflects, not only identifying the leading causes of death in infants, but the social, economic and health status of a country. Objective: The purpose of this study is to determine causes of under five mortality and provide an accurate estimate of child mortality rates as we transition from MDG to

---

* Correspondence: Kameel Mungrue, MBBS, MPH, FRIPH, MBA, Department of Paraclinical Sciences, Health and Primary Care, Faculty of Medical Sciences, University of the West Indies, Eric Williams Medical Sciences Complex, Mt. Hope, Trinidad. Email: kameel.mungrue@sta.uwi.edu.

SDG3. Design and methods: We created a database of deaths in children under 5 years in Trinidad from July 2013 to June 2014 from civil registration and vital statistics. This information was used to obtain the medical records for each death. Clinical details surrounding the birth and death of each death were extracted from the medical records, including date and cause of death. Results: Findings focused on gravidity, parity, type of death, APGAR score, maternal age, and birth weight. These factors were found to affect the risk of under-five mortality in Trinidad. The most common cause of death in under-five children was disorders relating to short gestation and unspecified low birth weight (ICD 10-P02). The under-five mortality rate was 18.4 per 1,000 live births. Conclusion: We provide evidence that short gestation and low birth weight (>1,500g) (ICD-10-PO2), and adolescent mothers were the main contributors to under five mortality. We also showed that an Apgar score did not identify babies most vulnerable.

INTRODUCTION

The World Summit for Children in 1990 (1), created an interest in measuring child mortality rates, both as a health indicator and as a fundamental measure of human development (2). Reduction of child mortality continues to attract global interest, partly due to the huge disparities between and within nations, and also by irrefutable proof that child mortality rates can be lowered even in resource-poor settings (3, 4). Several studies have reported a decline in child mortality among high-income, middle-income, and low-income countries (5-18). Thus the Millennium Development Goal 4 (MDG 4) target of reduction of child mortality by two thirds from 1990 to 2015 had wide support internationally (19-23). MDGs are well-defined quantifiable targets, which allow progress to be assessed within regions and countries. While it is predictable that this goal will not be realised by 2015, child mortality has since approximately halved, making these goals important contributors towards the progress of increased child survival (24-31). MDGs goals expired at the end of 2015 (31), and have been replaced by the Sustainable Development Goals (SDGs) to 2030. Although three of eight MDGs were devoted to health now only one of 17 SDGs represents all health issues. The new recommended targets include reducing neonatal mortality to at least 12 per 1,000 live births and under-5 mortality (U5MR) to 25 per 1,000 live births (32). Thus as we move from MDGs to SDG measuring progress hinges on current situational analysis guided by accurate data, particularly accurate causes of death to inform future policy responses.

Important gaps in our understanding of the drivers of mortality change, or what impedes progress requires continuous investigation. An evaluation of the dynamics of the relevant data related to child mortality is required to determine the level of progress as well as ascertain the necessary actions to be taken to achieve future goals. In this regard the MDG 4 target shifted the focus from tracking levels of child mortality to assessing whether countries are reducing child mortality at the 4.4% rate per year needed to achieve the two-thirds reduction in 25 years (33). Precise evaluations of rates of change call for more rigorous measurements particularly the collection of data relating to child mortality. Thus the most up to date, local, and valid assessments of trends in child mortality along with the associated drivers of these trends can provide an important input to national, regional, and global debates on next steps (33). Wang and colleagues recently showed that secular trend was the main explanatory variable attributable to child survival (34). Globally, social determinants, including socioeconomic and deeply rooted gender inequalities, remain important obstacles to child wellbeing (35). However rigorous assessments are needed to chart the way forward. If not, at minimum by 2030, 2.4 million children will die yearly (26), of which most would be neonatal deaths, an area most neglected. (36-38). Globally the proportion of neonatal deaths increased from 37% in 1990 to 44% in 2012 (39). Every year 11 million children are born in Latin American and the Caribbean of which 237,000 die by the first year and another 304,000 die before age five. Notwithstanding the region has seen significant reductions in infant mortality which has occurred faster than other regions (40). Trinidad and Tobago (TTO) is a small Anglophone Caribbean island situated just east of Venezuela. The most recent Ministry of Health (MoH) Annual Reports are for the period 2002-2004, which reported U5MRs of 27.4, 26.9, and 18.6 per 1,000 live births, IMRs of 24.2 24.0 16.5 per 1,000 live births and neonatal rates of 20.2 20.4 13.5 per 1,000 live births for these years (41). The leading causes of death among newborns in TT for the period 1998-2005 were pre-term births (less than 37 weeks gestation), severe infections, birth asphyxia, and congenital anomalies respectively (41). In comparison the most developed country in the region the USA has similar patterns. The top 5 causes of infant mortality in 2011 accounting for 58% of infant deaths were serious birth defects, underweight and preterm infants, sudden infant death syndrome (SIDS), maternal complications of pregnancy and injuries (42). Thus the purpose of this study is to determine causes of death in children under five and provide an estimate of child mortality rates as we approach the transition from MDG to SDG3.

OUR STUDY

The continuous registration of births and deaths through a system of civil registration and vital statistics (CRVS), is potentially the richest source of data about child mortality (43, 44). In TT by law (Births and Deaths Registration Act, Chap. 44:01) a medical certificate of the cause of death (MCCD) must be issued by the attending physician at the time of the death or within five days from the time of death except there is a coroner's investigation. In the absence of a physician or for medico legal issues a post mortem is performed to determine the cause of death prior to issuing the MCCD. Compliance with registration is almost complete as there are no reported cases of failure to report deaths especially in children. However there are occasional reports of indiscriminate disposal of fetuses and newborns. In this data set there is no sampling variance, though analysis may still be affected by small numbers of events. The MCCD is collected and forwarded to the Central Statistical Office (CSO) where it is stored and a death certificate in turn is issued which is used for the disposal of the dead. The starting point for the study was a review of the MCCD collected and stored at the CSO. The MCCD has a registration number, the age at death, the causes of death and the location where the death occurred. This information was extracted and used to create a database of mortality in children = 5 years in Trinidad from July 2013 to June 2014. We used this information to locate and obtain the medical records for each death. We reviewed each record and cross checked the data in the medical records with the MCCD issued to validate the age and cause of each death and to obtain other clinical parameters. Further questions were designed and adapted using the 2012 WHO verbal autopsy instrument to guide the process (45). The data collected included birth weight, gravidity, parity, APGAR score (only performed at 1-minute i.e., 1-min APGAR), maternal age and cause of death. We used the single category 15-19 years to define adolescent pregnancies and did not use separate age groups, such as <15-year-olds, 16–17-years, and 18–19-years because of the small numbers. We used the WHO definitions for live birth and infant death but perinatal death as occurring up to 7 days after birth (45). We defined low birth weight as <2,500gm based on the WHO classification (46). We restricted our study to two large teaching hospitals the Mount Hope Maternity Hospital (MHMH) in the north of the island and the San Fernando General Hospital (SFGH) in the south, which provides a larger population as well as it offers the opportunity to compare areas. The mortality rate was calculated by the number of deaths among children under five years per 1,000 live births. The cause-specific mortality rate was calculated by the number of deaths among children under 5 years of age caused by a specific disease per 1000 live births.

The ICD-10 codes were used to classify each death (47). This data were used to calculate relevant mortality rates for the period of study with 95% confidence intervals (CI). All test were two tailed and significance is reported at p = 0.05. All data was stored and analyzed using SPSS vs16. Ethical approval for study was obtained from the University of the West Indies Ethics Committee and all other relevant stakeholders.

Our Findings

We identified 345 deaths from the MCCD for the period under study and reported an U5MR of 18.8 per 1,000 live births (95% CI 16.8-20.4) for the one year period July 2013 –June 2014 and a neonatal mortality rate of 3.5 per 1,000 live births. This represents the most accurate estimate of under five year mortality in Trinidad. Cause-specific mortality derived from the MCCD was classified using the ICD-10 classification, see Table 1. The top five causes of death in children under five years of age were 1) low birth weight (PO2), 56 (16.2%), 2) disorders relating to length of gestation and foetal growth (P05-P08), 47 (13.6), 3) septicemia (A40-A41) 25 (7.2%) and respiratory conditions (P22), 25 (7.2%), and respiratory distress syndrome (P20-P21) 24(7%) (see Table 5). An important finding was HIV was not a contributing factor to under-five mortality, possible due to HIV screening of all antenatal mothers and the effective use of antiretroviral agents in preventing mother to child transmission (48).

Table 1. Cause-specific mortality based on reported immediate cause of death on MCCD, classified using ICD-10 codes

Cause of death	n(%)
Gastrointestinal diseases (K 50-54, K 29), A04, A08, A09 A02.2)	5(1.4)
Septicemia (A40-A41)	25(7.2)
Pneumonia & influenza (J10-J18)	5(1.5)
Remainder of infectious diseases & parasite(A00-A01, A02.1-A03, A05-A07, A-16-A39, A42-49, B00-B99	5(1.5)
Congenital Malformations, Deformities & chromosomal abnormalities (Q00-Q99)	14(4.1)
Low birth weight (P02)	56(16.3)
Disorders relating to length of gestation and foetal growth (P05-P08)	47(13.6)
Intrauterine hypoxia and birth hypoxia (P10-P15)	5(1.5)
Respiratory distress syndrome (P20- P21)	24(7)
Other respiratory conditions (P22)	25(7.2)
Neonatal Haemorrhage (P35-P39)	10(2.8)
Sudden Infant death syndrome (P29, P70-P83)	1(0.3)
Unintentional Injury (R95)	1(0.3)
Ill-defined and unspecified (R99)	122(35.4)
Total	345(100)

Table 2. The distribution of under 5 mortality by perinatal (0-7 days), neonatal (8-27days), and infants 28 days- 1 year and children >1- ≤5 years (yrs.) mortalities for the periods July 2013 to December 2013 and January 2014 to June 2014, and for the one year continuous period

Category of Death	July	Aug	Sept	Oct	Nov	Dec	Total n(%)	Jan	Feb	Mar	Apr	May	June	Total n(%)	One year n(%)
Perinatal	1	3	2	8	3	6	23(48)	4	4	1	1	5	2	17(38)	40(43)}*
Neonatal	1	1	1	3	7	0	36(27)	1	2	0	2	2	5	29(27)	65(27)
Infant	3	1	1	2	2	2	11(23)	4	3	3	0	1	5	16 (35)	27(29)
0-5	1	0	0	0	0	0	1(2)	0	0	0	0	0	0	0(0)	1(1)
Total	6	5	4	13	12	7	48(100)	9	9	4	3	8	9	45(100)	93(100)

* Perinatal deaths included in neonatal deaths.

Further analysis showed that 142 deaths occurred at the MHMH and 153 occurred at the SFGH hence there was no significant difference in the counts from the two geographical areas. This also means that 295 of the 345 deaths or 86% of deaths occurred at theses two institutions. Hence all other intuitions not studied contributed to only 14% to the age under 5 years mortality. Of the 142 deaths occurring at the MHMH only 52 (37%) medical records were available for review, similarly only 41 of the 153 (29%) deaths at SFGH were also available for review. Therefore we only reviewed 93 (27%) of deaths that occurred, Table 2. The main reasons were some records were inadequate as they provided no relevant information, others were handwritten and difficult to discern and missing records. Perinatal deaths accounted for the majority (48% and 38%) of under-five mortality, while there was only one death in the age group 1-5 years.

A significantly higher proportion of deaths ($p<0.05$) occurred in children with a 1-min Apgar score of 9-7 (36, 38.7%) than children with a score of 0-3 (16, 17.02%), Table 3. Mothers in the age group 15-19 had the highest rate (1.6 per 1000 live births) of under-five mortality (see Table 4) and 52% of under-5 deaths occurred in mothers who were either in their first or second pregnancy, see Table 5.

Table 3. Distribution of 1-min Apgar scores for the period July 2013 to June 2014, among the 93 infant deaths reviewed

	Jul-Dec 2013	Jan-Jun 2014	Year Total
Apgar	n(%)	n(%)	n(%)
9-7	15(30)	21(48.8)	36(38.7)
6	7(14)	3(7)	10(10.8)
5	4(8)	4(9.3)	8(8.5)
4	8(16)	6(14)	14(15.1)
0-3	11(22)	5(11.6)	16(17.2)
Not recorded	5(10)	4(9.3)	9(9.7)
Total	50(100)	43(100)	93(100)

Table 4. The distribution of under-5 mortality by maternal ages for the period July 2013 to June 2014

	2013 Jul-Dec	2014 Jan-Jun		Number of Live births	Under-5 mortality per 1000 live births by maternal age
Maternal Age	n(%)	n(%)	Total		
15-19	6(12)	2(4.65)	8	490	16.3
20-24	5(10)	8(18.6)	13	3499	3.7
25-29	14(28)	12(26.67)	26	5388	5.0
30-34	10(20)	10(23.26)	20	4441	4.5
≥35	10(20)	11(25.58)	21	2913	7.2
Unknown	5(10)	0(0)	5		
Total	50(100)	43(100)	93		

Table 5. Maternal gravidity and under-five mortality for the period July 2013 to June 2014

	2013	2014	
Gravidity	n(%)	n(%)	Total
1	11(22)	11(25.6)	22
2	15(30)	12(27.9)	27
3	8(16)	9(20.9)	17
4	4(8)	4(9.3)	7
5	2(4)	0(0.00)	2
>5	3(6)	1(2.3)	4
Unknown	7(14)	6(14)	14
Total	50(100)	43(100)	93

The majority 58 (62.3%) of deaths occurred among babies with a LBW. There was a very strong negative correlation (R2 = -0.9) between and under-5 deaths and birth weight.

Discussion

We report an U5MR rate of 18.8 per 1,000 live births for the one year period July 2013-June 2014, which is below the SDG goal of 25 per 1000 live births. Progress has been made as reflected by declining rates of U5MRs as reported both by the MoH (27.4, 26.9, and 18.6 per 1,000 live births) for the period 2002-2004 and the UN Inter-agency Group for Child Mortality (31, 29, and 20 per, 1000 live births in 1990, 2000, and 2015), which realized an annual rate of reduction of 1.6% (41, 49). However our study shows that the downward trend has plateaued and there was a marginal increase in U5MR. Hence we did not achieve the Millennium Development Goal 4, which called for an annual rate of reduction of the U5MR of 4.4% between 1990 and 2015. Under five mortality is an important indicator of child health and overall development of a nation, as it reflects the social, economic, and environmental conditions in which children (and others in society) live, including the healthcare system (50). Although the U5MR reported in this study is three times higher than the average rate in high-income countries (6-7 deaths per 1,000 live births) it is four times better than African countries (81 per 1,000 live births (51).

The leading cause of the under five year mortality was low birth weight (cause specific mortality rate 3 per 1,000 live births. Worldwide an estimated 20 million babies are born with LBW each year and contribute to 60-80% of neonatal deaths, 95.5% of which occur in developing countries (52). Hence the results of this study i.e., 60% of under-5 mortality was associated with LBW support claims that 60-80% of children born with LBW are more likely to die. In addition it also supports the previous MDG strategy for reducing child mortality; which states that the global percentage of LBW infants born per year should be estimated despite the fact that >50% of newborns are not weighed at birth (53). The reduction of low birth weight must therefore play a pivotal role in reducing child mortality in the future. The first steps must focus on improving perinatal services and the quality of neonatal intensive care both of which have been shown to impact on LBW (54, 55). In our study, the second highest cause of death was due to Septicemia (25, 27%) (ICD A40-A41). The World

Health Organization (WHO) estimates that 1 million deaths per year (10% of all under-five mortality) are due to neonatal sepsis (56).

The highest rates of septicemia occur in premature, low-birth-weight (LBW) infants and those with depressed function at birth, as manifested by a low Apgar score (57). Another important contributor to under-5 mortality is respiratory distress syndrome (RDS), which was associated with a quarter (25.8%) of all deaths a finding consistent with others (58).

The Apgar score was designed to provide a mechanism to record fetal to neonatal transitioning (59, 60), the probability of survival of the infant, and to appraise the need for resuscitation. Regrettable only 1-min APGAR scores were recorded and available for analysis. We found that mortality was highest (30%) among neonates with a 1-min APGAR of 9-7. As far back as 1964 Drage and colleagues (61) showed that neonates with low scores at 5 minutes had an increase probability of dying over neonates with low 1-min scores. More recently Fei Li and colleagues (62) showed that the 5-min Apgar score is a good and convenient predictor of infant death. However, The American Academy of Pediatrics and the American College of Obstetricians and Gynecologists in their most recent statement (63) stated that the Apgar score "does not predict individual neonatal mortality or neurologic outcome, and should not be used for that purpose" (64). In addition it also states that, "A 1-minute Apgar score of 0–3 does not predict any individual infant's outcome" (64). The high percentage of deaths (30%) with an APGAR score of 7-9 at 1-minute and a lower percentage of deaths (17.2%) in babies with a low APGAR score support both recommendations (65).

A critical finding of the study is adolescent childbearing, had the highest mortality (16.3 per 1,000 live births) 4.4 times higher than the maternal age group 20-25 years. Donoso et al. (66) in Chile reported that the maternal age 20-29 years was associated with the lowest risk of maternal, fetal, neonatal and infant mortality. The consequences of this finding are many. Firstly the recognition that the risks associated adolescent childbearing in the developing world continues to be a major challenge. Secondly the consequences of an unplanned teenage pregnancy are both short term and long term. The latter include psychosocial issues such as life goals and financial stability, attaining higher educational levels, marital instability and difficulty regulating family size (63-65). In addition short-term consequences include poor obstetric care and poor birth outcomes (51), including very preterm and preterm delivery, low birth weight (67), small for gestational age and the experience and characteristics of the youngest mothers (58). It is evident that confronting childbearing in this vulnerable age group can contribute to improving child survival.

LIMITATIONS

This study has some intrinsic limitations. The data are retrospective and in a third of all the deaths the medical reports were not retrievable. Emphasizing that even where vital statistics are collected and death certification is a legal requirement, data in developing countries are poorly stored and therefore may become unavailable or difficult to access. Medical records that can be retrieved are hand written and sometimes illegible. Hence a Children Death Report System as part of a national surveillance system is strongly recommended. The study is cross-sectional in nature and hence casualty cannot be established. We were constrained by the information included in the vital statistics registry and, therefore, were not able to examine the social determinants such as sociodemographic, financial, or personal information that may have affected birth outcomes. The strength of the study is in 27% of the deaths we were able to follow from birth to death.

In conclusion we provide evidence that short gestation, low birth weight (>1,500g) (ICD-10-PO2), and adolescent mothers were the main contributors to under 5 years of age mortality. We also showed that an Apgar score did not identify babies most vulnerable. These results will be useful for the Ministry of Health to inform appropriate strategies to reduce under five mortality in the future.

REFERENCES

[1] United Nations. World declaration on the survival, protection and development of children and plan of action for implementing the world declaration on the survival, protection and development of children in the 1990s: World summit for children. 1990. New York: UN Publications. URL: http://www.unicef.org/wsc/plan.htm.

[2] Murray CJ, Laakso T, Shibuya K, Hill K, Lopez AD. Can we achieve Millennium Development Goal 4? New analysis of country trends and forecasts of under-5 mortality to 2015. Lancet 2007;370:1040-54.

[3] Jones G, Steketee RW, Black RE, Bhutta ZA, Morris SS, for the Bellagio Child Survival Study Group. How many child deaths can we prevent this year? Lancet 2003;362:65-71.

[4] Lawn JE, Kerber K, Enweronu-Laryea C, Massee Bateman O. Newborn survival in low resource settings--are we delivering? BJOG 2009;116(Suppl 1):49-59.

[5] Rajaratnam JK, Marcus JR, Flaxman AD, Wang H, Layghn-Rector A, Dwyer l, et al. Neonatal, postneonatal, childhood, and under-5 mortality for 187 countries, 1970—2010: A systematic analysis of progress towards Millennium Development Goal 4. Lancet 2010;375:1988-2008.

[6] Lozano R, Wang H, Foreman KJ, Rajaratnam JK, Naghavi M, Marcus Jr, et al. Progress towards Millennium Development Goals 4 and 5 on maternal and child mortality: An updated systematic analysis. Lancet 2011;378:1139-65.

[7] Hill K, You D, Inoue M, Oestergaard MZ, for the Technical Advisory Group of United Nations Inter-agency Group for Child Mortality Estimation. Child mortality estimation: accelerated progress in reducing global child mortality, 1990—2010. PLoS Med 2012;9: e1001303.

[8] United Nations Department of International Economic and Social Affairs. Mortality of children under age 5: World estimates and projections, 1950—2025. Herndon, VA: United Nations, 1988.

[9] Hill K, Amouzou A. Trends in child mortality, 1960 to 2000. In: Jamison DT, Feachem RG, Makgoba MW, eds. Disease and mortality in Sub-Saharan Africa. Washington, DC: World Bank, 2006.

[10] Wang H, Dwyer-Lindgren L, Lofgren KT, Rajaratnam JK, Marcus JR, Levin-RectorA, et al. Age-specific and sex-specific mortality in 187 countries, 1970-2010: A systematic analysis for the Global Burden of Disease Study 2010. Lancet 2012;380:2071-94.

[11] Alkema L, You D. Child mortality estimation: a comparison of UN IGME and IHME estimates of levels and trends in under-five mortality rates and deaths. PLoS Med 2012; 9:e1001288.

[12] Guillot M, Gerland P, Pelletier F, Saabneh A. Child mortality estimation: a global overview of infant and child mortality age patterns in light of new empirical data. PLoS Med 2012;9:e1001299.

[13] Doces JA. Democracy and child mortality: can we claim causality? Yes, but it's indirect. URL: http://citation.allacademic.com/meta/p_mla_apa_research_citation/1/9/7/3/2/p197328_index.html.

[14] Franco A, Alvarez-Dardet C, Ruiz MT. Effect of democracy on health: ecological study. BMJ 2004;329:1421-3.

[15] Lazarova EA. Governance in relation to infant mortality rate: evidence from around the world. Ann Public Coop Econ 2006;77:385-94.

[16] Lena HF, London B. The political and economic determinants of health outcomes: a cross-national analysis. Int J Health Serv 1993;23:585-602.

[17] Navia P, Zweifel TD. Democracy, dictatorship, and infant mortality revisited. J Democracy 2003;14:90-103.

[18] Shandra JM, Nobles J, London B, Williamson JB. Dependency, democracy, and infant mortality: a quantitative, cross-national analysis of less developed countries. Soc Sci Med 2004;59:321-33.

[19] Zweifel TD, Navia P. Democracy, dictatorship, and infant mortality. J Democracy 2000; 11:99-114.

[20] UNICEF. Committing to child survival: A promise renewed. Progress report 2013. New York: United Nations Children's Fund, 2013.

[21] Secretary-General UN. Integrated and coordinated implementation of and follow-up to the outcomes of the major United Nations conferences and summits in the economic, social and related fields: report of the Secretary-General. New York: United Nations, 2004.

[22] USAID. Child survival: call to action. Ending preventable child deaths. URL: http://5thbday.usaid.gov/pages/responsesub/roadmap.pdf.

[23] GAVI Alliance. Investing in immunisation through the GAVI Alliance. URL: http://www.gavialliance.org/library/publications/the-evidence-base/investing-in-immunisation-through-the-gavi-alliance-the-evidence-base/.

[24] WHO. Monitoring maternal, newborn and child health: Understanding key progress indicators. URL: http://www.who.int/healthmetrics/news/monitoring_maternal_newborn_child_health.pdf.

[25] UNICEF. Monitoring the situation of children and women. URL: http://data.unicef.org/about.

[26] Wang H, Liddell CA, Coates MM, Mooney MD, Levitz CE, Schumacher AE, et al. Global, regional, and national levels of neonatal, infant, and under-5 mortality during 1990–2013: A systematic analysis for the Global Burden of Disease Study 2013. Lancet 2014;384(9947):957–79.

[27] WHO, UNICEF, UNFPA, The World Bank, United Nations Population Division. Trends in maternal mortality: 1990 to 2013. Estimates by WHO, UNICEF, UNFPA, The World Bank and the United Nations Population Division. Geneva: World Health Organization, 2014.

[28] Kassebaum NJ, Bertozzi-Villa A, Coggeshall MS, Shackelford KA, Steiner C, Heuton KR, et al. Global, regional, and national levels and causes of maternal

mortality during 1990—2013: A systematic analysis for the Global Burden of Disease Study 2013. Lancet 2014;384(9947):980-1004.

[29] Liu L, Johnson HL, Cousens S, Perin J, Scott S, Lawn JE, et al. Global, regional, and national causes of child mortality: An updated systematic analysis for 2010 with time trends since 2000. Lancet 2012;379:2151-61.

[30] Norheim O, Jha P, Admasu K, Godal T, Hum R, Kruk M, et al. Avoiding 40% of the premature deaths in each country, 2010–30: Review of national mortality trends to help quantify the UN Sustainable Development Goal for health. Lancet 2015;385(9964):239-52.

[31] Rohde J, Cousens S, Chopra M, Tangcharoensathien V, Black R, Bhutta ZA, et al. 30 years after Alma-Ata: Has primary health care worked in countries? Lancet 2008;372(9642):950-61.

[32] Open Working Group. Outcome Document—Open Working Group on Sustainable Development Goals. URL: http://sustainabledevelopment.un.org/focussdgs.html.

[33] United Nations Sustainable Development Goals. URL: http://www.un.org/sustainabledevelopment/sustainable-development-goals.

[34] Rajaratnam J, Marcus J, Flaxman A, Wang H, Levin-Rector A, Dwyer L, et al. Neonatal, postneonatal, childhood, and under-5 mortality for 187 countries, 1970–2010: A systematic analysis of progress towards Millennium Development Goal 4. Lancet 2010;375(9730):1988-2008.

[35] Wang H, Liddell C, Coates M, Mooney M, Levitz C, Schumacher A, et al. Global, regional, and national levels of neonatal, infant, and under-5 mortality during 1990–2013: A systematic analysis for the Global Burden of Disease Study 2013. Lancet 2014;384(9947):957-79.

[36] Yuan B, Målqvist M, Trygg N, Qian X, Ng N, Thomsen S. What interventions are effective on reducing inequalities in maternal and child health in low- and middle-income settings? A systematic review. BMC Public Health 2014;14:634.

[37] UNICEF. Levels and trends in child mortality. New York: United Nations, 2013. URL: http://www.childinfo.org/files/Child_Mortality_Report_2013.pdf.

[38] Lawn JE, Kinney M, Black RE, Pitt C, Cousens S, Kerber K, et al. A decade of change for newborn survival, policy and programmes: a multi-country analysis. Health Policy Plan 2012;27(Suppl 3):6-28.

[39] Lawn JE, Blencowe H, Oza S, You D, lee ACC, Waiswa P, et al. Every newborn: Progress, priorities, potential beyond survival. Lancet 2014. doi.org/10.1016/S0140-6736(14)60496-7.

[40] Darmstadt G, Marchant T, Claeson M, Brown W, Morris S, Donnay F, et al. A strategy for reducing maternal and newborn deaths by 2015 and beyond. BMC Pregnancy Childbirth 2013;13(1):216.

[41] Cepal.org. Millenium Development Goals Fact Sheet Goal 4: Reduce the under-five mortality rate, 2010. URL: http://www.cepal.org/MDG/noticias/paginas/6/40006/MDG4_CHILD_MORTALITY_FACT_SHEET.pdf.

[42] The Government of Trinidad and Tobago, University of West Indies (HEU) and UNICEF. Situation analysis of children and women in Trinidad and Tobago, 2010.
[43] Infant mortality: Maternal and infant health.Reproductive health, 2014. URL: http://www.cdc.gov/reproductivehealth/maternalinfanthealth/infantmortality.htm
[44] AbouZahr, C, de Savigny, D, Mikkelsen L, Setel PW, Lozano R, Nichol E, et al. Civil registration and vital statistics: progress in the data revolution for counting and accountability. Lancet 2015. doi.org/10.1016/S0140-6736(15)60173-8.
[45] The 2012 WHO verbal autopsy instrument. Geneva: World Health Organization, 2012.
[46] Phillips DE, AbouZahr C, Lopez AD, Mikkelsen L, de Savigny D, Lozano R, et al. Are well functioning civil registration and vital statistics systems associated with better health outcomes? Lancet 2015;386;1373-75.
[47] International statistical classification of diseases and related health problems, Tenth revision (ICD-10), Vol 2. Geneva: World Health Organization; 2006.
[48] Mungrue K. Monitoring the effectiveness of prevention of mother-to-child (MTCT) HIV transmission in Trinidad a small middle income country, 2013-2016. J Prev Treat HIV/AIDS 2017;2(1):1-4.
[49] UN Inter-agency Group for Child Mortality Estimation. Levels and trends in Child mortality report 2015. URL: unicef.org
[50] McGuire JW. Basic health care provision and under-5 mortality: A cross-national study of developing countries. World Dev 2006;34(3):405–25.
[51] Katz J, West KP, Khatry SK, Christian P, LeClerq, Pradhan EK, et al. Risk factors for early infant mortality in Sarlahi District, Nepal. Bull World Health Organ 2003;81(10):717-25.
[52] World Health Organization. Care of the preterm/low birth weight newborn. URL: http://www.who.int/maternal_child_adolescent/topics/newborn/care_of_preterm/en/
[53] The United Nations Children's Fund and World Health Organization. Low birth weight. Country regional and global estimates. Geneva: WHO, 2004.
[54] Corchia C, Orzalesi M. Geographic variations in outcome of very low birth weight infants in Italy. Acta Paediatr 2007;96(1):35-8.
[55] World Health Organization, Report. Global Health Observatory (GHO), data. 2015. URL: http://www.who.int/gho/child_health/mortality/mortality_under_five_text/en/]
[56] WHO Statistical Information Systems (WHOSIS), 2011. URL: http://www.who.int/whosis/indicators/compendium/2008/2bwn/en/index.html.
[57] Lawn J, Cousens S, Zupan J. 4 million neonatal deaths: When? Where? Why? Lancet 2005;365(9462):891-900.
[58] Edmond K, Zaidi A. New approaches to preventing, diagnosing, and treating neonatal sepsis. PLoS Med 2010;7(3):e1000213
[59] Kamath B, MacGuire E, McClure E, Goldenberg R, Jobe A. Neonatal mortality from respiratory distress syndrome: Lessons for low-resource countries. Pediatrics 2011;127(6):1139-46.

[60] The Apgar score. Committee Opinion No. 644. American College of Obstetricians and Gynecologists. Obstet Gynecol 2015;126:e52–5.

[61] Drage JS Kennedy C, Schwarz BK. The apgar score as an index of neonatal mortality. a report from the collaborative study of cerebral palsy. Obstet Gynecol 1964;24:222-30.

[62] Li F, Wu T, Lei X, Zhang H, Mao M, Zhang J. The Apgar Score and Infant Mortality. PLoS One 2013;8(7):e69072. doi:10.1371/journal.pone.0069072.

[63] Card JJ, Wise LL. Teenage mothers and teenage fathers: The impact of early childbearing on the parents' personal and professional lives. Fam Plann Perspect 1978;10:199–205.

[64] Rathod S, Singh M, Damor R, Jankar D, Gosalia V, Patel H, et al. Socio-demographic profile of infant mortality by verbal autopsy in urban area of Bhavnagar, Gujarat. J Commun Med 2011;2(3):1.

[65] Agrawal A, Kumar R, Kumar P. Early neonatal mortality in a hilly North Indian State: Socio demographic factor and treatment seeking behaviour. Indian J Prev Soc Med 2003(34);46-51.

[66] Donoso E, Carvajal JA, Vera C, Poblete JA. Women age as a risk factor for maternal, fetal, neonatal and infant mortality. Rev Méd Chile 2014;142(2):168-74.

[67] Corchia C, Orzalesi M. Geographic variations in outcome of very low birth weight infants in Italy. Acta Paediatr 2007;96(1):35-8.

In: Childhood and Adolescence
Editor: Joav Merrick

ISBN: 978-1-53613-574-9

Chapter 5

TRAINING OF POTENTIAL PROGRAM IMPLEMENTERS FOR THE TIN KA PING P.A.T.H.S. PROJECT IN CHINA: SUBJECTIVE OUTCOME EVALUATION FINDINGS

Daniel TL Shek*[1-6,*]*, PhD, FHKPS, BBS, SBS, JP, Janet TY Leung*[1]*, PhD, Lawrence K Ma*[1]*, PhD, Li Lin*[1]*, PhD and Florence KY Wu*[1]*, EdD

[1]Department of Applied Social Sciences, The Hong Kong Polytechnic University, Hong Kong, PR China
[2]Centre for Innovative Programmes for Adolescents and Families, The Hong Kong Polytechnic University, Hong Kong, PR China
[3]Department of Social Work, East China Normal University, Shanghai, PR China
[4]Kiang Wu Nursing College of Macau, Macau, PR China

[*] Correspondence: Daniel TL Shek, PhD, FHKPS, BBS, SBS, JP, Associate Vice President (Undergraduate Programme) and Chair Professor of Applied Social Sciences, Department of Applied Social Sciences, The Hong Kong Polytechnic University, Hunghom, Hong Kong, PR China. E-mail: daniel.shek@polyu.edu.hk.

[5]Hong Kong Institute of Service Leadership and Management Limited, Hong Kong, PR China
[6]Division of Adolescent Medicine, Department of Pediatrics, Kentucky Children's Hospital, University of Kentucky School of Medicine, Lexington, Kentucky, USA

Utilizing the subjective outcome evaluation approach, the present study examined the views of the potential program implementers of the Tin Ka Ping P.A.T.H.S. Project held in Jiujiang, China. Upon completion of this workshop, a total of 171 junior and senior secondary school colleagues completed a well-validated close-ended questionnaire by rating on dimensions including training content, instructor quality, administrative arrangements, and perceived self-performance. Analyses revealed that an overwhelming proportion of trainees indicated satisfaction with all these four dimensions. Echoing the previous findings, perceived training quality significantly predicted participants' perceived benefits and overall satisfaction. Instructor quality also significantly predicted perceived benefits, with the latter being a significant predictor of overall satisfaction as well. In conjunction with other studies assessing the effectiveness of the training workshops, the present evaluation study indicates that the training workshops of the Tin Ka Ping P.A.T.H.S. Project are positively perceived by the potential program implementers.

INTRODUCTION

While globalization underscored the remarkable economic ascension of China in the past few decades (1, 2), concerns have been raised regarding its negative impact on the mental health status of Chinese people (3). Particularly, Bhat and Rather (4) outlined how globalization had vicariously led to a worsened mental well-being of Chinese youth via the increased educational competitions and parental demands to excel. Specifically, findings from a cross-provincial study by the National Institute of Education Sciences (NIES) revealed that 47.39% of the Chinese students thought their parents were unreasonably harsh, and 63.21% indicated the desire for parents' encouragement and recognition (5). Meanwhile, 60.59% of the surveyed parents opined that they would prioritize their children's academic achievement over crucial developmental facets like character formation and interpersonal communications, but only around three-tenths of these parents indicated satisfaction with their children's academic performance.

As family plays an important role in adolescent development, the Ministry of Education (6) publicized five recommendations on how to optimize family education. One major strategy entails the provision of a healthy, enriching living habitat which permits the positive emotional and physical development of adolescents. While these guidelines appear comprehensive, findings from the NIES (5) study clearly suggested that more has to be done in the school context. In conjunction with the absence of systematic teaching resources imperative for implementing mental health education in China (7), there is a call for the initiation of positive youth development (PYD) programs aimed at strengthening the psychosocial competences in Chinese adolescents. Echoing the recommendation by the Ministry of Education, Damon (8) argued that PYD approach centers upon the person-in-environment and strength-based principles. Rather than combating a specific youth issue, the PYD approach constitutes the prevention of a barrage of adolescent problems through the nurturance of adolescents' talents, strengths, and potentials (8).

With respect to other Chinese communities, Shek and colleagues (9) remarked that over the years, youngsters in Hong Kong have also shown problems such as internet addiction, materialism, and adolescent premarital sex. Against such a backdrop, a multi-year PYD project entitled "Positive Adolescent Training through Holistic Social Programs" (Project P.A.T.H.S.), financed by The Hong Kong Jockey Club Charities Trust and tailored for junior secondary students in Hong Kong, was launched in 2005. The two-tier Project P.A.T.H.S. targeted both the general junior secondary student population (i.e., Tier 1 Program) and the adolescents with greater psychosocial needs (i.e., Tier 2 Program). Findings from a multitude of evaluation studies corroborated the effectiveness of the Project P.A.T.H.S. in promoting holistic adolescent development in Hong Kong (10, 11).

Despite the unprecedented success of the Project P.A.T.H.S. in Hong Kong, one may ask whether the project can be successfully replicated in other Chinese communities (12). With the financial support of Tin Ka Ping Foundation, the pilot phase of the project entitled "Tin Ka Ping Positive Adolescent Training through Holistic Social Program" (Tin Ka Ping P.A.T.H.S. Project) was launched in four schools in East China (namely, Changzhou, Shanghai, Suzhou, and Yangzhou) from 2011 to 2014. Findings from multiple evaluation studies (12, 13) showed the promise of the project. Consequently, the second phase was launched in the academic year 2014-2015 as the preparatory year, followed by the full-implementation phase involving over 30 secondary schools in mainland China in the subsequent three academic years (14).

Similar to other PYD programs, the Tin Ka Ping P.A.T.H.S. Project emphasizes systematic training incorporating elements of experiential and reflective learning. Accordingly, similar to previous train-the-trainer programs conducted during the preparatory year (15), prospective implementers were expected to assume the role as students and actively engage in each training session. Experience sharing on teaching methods, opportunities to self-reflect, and discussion about one's views on the various PYD constructs were heavily featured in previous training workshops conducted in East China (see 14).

In the academic year 2016-2017, three training workshops targeting prospective implementers of the Tin Ka Ping P.A.T.H.S. Project were scheduled to take place in Jiujiang (in Jiangxi Province), Shijiazhuang (in Hebei Province), and Baiyin (in Gansu Province). This chapter features primarily the analyses of participants' perception of the first workshop held in Jiujiang in December 2016. Information about the schedules and major activities of the training workshop are detailed in the Appendix. Through this 2.5-day train-the-trainer program, there were several objectives that we endeavored to achieve: i) consolidation of participants' grasps of the concepts and rationale of PYD; ii) promotion of trainees' understanding and positive attitude toward adolescent development; iii) familiarization of participants with the design, rationale, execution, and evaluation of the Tin Ka Ping P.A.T.H.S. Project; iv) strengthening participants' understanding of the content and activities developed for the project; v) facilitation of participants' reflection and acquisition of the appropriate mentality, knowledge, and teaching skills instrumental to the successful implementation of the project and; vi) establishment of a self-help network among the trainees.

As remarked by Clarke (16), in-service training is instrumental to the effective functioning of a human service program. Echoing Clarke's (16) notion, Shek and colleagues (17, 18) outlined five elements crucial to the success of every PYD program, including people, place, policy, process, and program (i.e., "5Ps"). Amongst them, the factor "people," argued to be the most influential factor, covers both implementers and participants of the program. As a result, the provision of quality on-site training to prospective implementers is indispensable to the successful implementation of the Tin Ka Ping P.A.T.H.S. Project. Furthermore, Kirkpatrick's (19) Four-Level (i.e., reaction, learning, behavior, and results) Training Evaluation Model underlined the necessity to empirically examine the effectiveness of any training programs. Indeed, several training evaluation studies utilizing the client satisfaction approach were administered in the preparatory year (14) and in the academic year 2015-2016 (20, 21) of the Tin Ka Ping P.A.T.H.S. Project, and the results have been hugely encouraging.

Because of the geographical and socioeconomic differences within mainland China, it is necessary to look at the impact of different training programs for the Tin Ka Ping P.A.T.H.S. Project. Therefore, utilizing the subjective outcome evaluation approach, the present study attempted to look into the effectiveness of the Tin Ka Ping P.A.T.H.S. Project training workshop held in Jiujiang in December 2016. Particularly, there were several research questions in this study:

1) What are the views of the program participants on the different aspects of the training program? Based on previous findings (15, 22), we predicted that a high proportion of the participants would

have positive perceptions of the program attributes (i.e., Hypothesis 1).

2) Are different aspects of the subjective outcome evaluation related to one another? Based on previous studies (15, 22, 23), we predicted that there would be significant correlations amongst all different dimensions of the present workshop, including training content, instructor quality, and administrative arrangements (i.e., Hypotheses 2a to 2f).
3) What constitute the predictors of participants' perceived benefits of the workshop? Based on previous findings (20, 23), we hypothesized that perceived training quality, instructor quality, administrative arrangements and self-performance would be significant predictors (i.e., Hypotheses 3a to 3d).
4) Would trainees' perceptions of the workshop (training quality, instructor quality, administrative arrangements, overall benefits, and self-performance) predict their overall satisfaction with the present train-the-trainer program? With reference to previous findings (22, 23), we hypothesized that all these dimensions would be significantly predictive of participants' overall satisfaction measure (i.e., Hypotheses 4a to 4e).

OUR STUDY

In the academic year 2016-2017, the first train-the-trainer workshop of the Tin Ka Ping P.A.T.H.S. Project was held in Jiujiang, China with a duration of 2.5 days. A total of 199 professionals from 39 institutions including secondary schools, non-governmental organizations, and universities participated in the study.

By the end of the workshop, we invited all participants to fill out a subjective outcome evaluation survey examining their views on the training workshop. Nonetheless, some of them did not participate as they left the workshop earlier due to transportation constraints. Altogether 171 questionnaires were returned to the Research Team. Amongst them, 62 were males (36.3%) and 109 were females (63.7%). Apart from nine respondents who selected social workers or the option 'others' as their occupations, the rest (N= 162, 94.74%) were teachers with 86 teaching at junior secondary schools and 76 working at senior secondary schools. The average work experience was 13.13 (SD: 8.71) years.

Instruments

The subjective outcome evaluation (SOE) questionnaire was utilized to solicit the trainees' feedback (via rating on a 5-point Likert Scale ranging from "strongly disagree" to "strongly agree") on several key components of the training workshop. Particularly, the quantitative part of the SOE questionnaire (SOE scale hereafter with 31 close-ended items) measures the following dimensions:

1) Participants' satisfaction with the training content (16 items). This included perceived benefits (9 items), training quality (5 items) and the overall satisfaction measures (2 items).
2) Participants' evaluations of the instructors (5 items), including the perceived good mastery of the curriculum and clarity of teaching.
3) Participants' perceptions of the administrative arrangements (6 items), including the workshops' location and reception provided by the training team.
4) Participants' evaluation of their own performance during the training (4 items), such as active participation in discussion and enhanced confidence to implement a program.

The SOE scale, which was utilized in previous Project P.A.T.H.S. train-the-trainer workshops conducted in Hong Kong (e.g., 24, 25) and mainland China (e.g., 15, 22, 23), has been repeatedly shown to possess excellent internal consistencies (i.e., Cronbach's alphas > 0.9). While the SOE questionnaire also comprises two open-ended questions on trainees' views on areas that warrant improvement and those that are praise-worthy, the present analysis is primarily focused on the analyses of the quantitative part (i.e., the SOE scale).

FINDINGS

Reliability analyses underscored the excellent internal consistency of the SOE scale (see Table 1). While the entire scale (31 items) yielded the highest Cronbach's alpha value ($\alpha = 0.95$), subscales on training content (16 items, $\alpha = 0.92$), instructor quality (5 items, $\alpha = 0.92$), perceived self-performance (4 items, $\alpha = 0.79$), and the administrative arrangements of the workshop (6 items, $\alpha = 0.87$) all displayed meritorious reliability.

The mean ratings on all subscales were over 4.00 with 5.00 being the maximum, indicating the overall participant satisfaction with the various dimensions of the training workshop. Multivariate analysis of variance (MANOVA) was adopted to examine if the satisfaction ratings differed across the senior and junior secondary school colleagues. Apart from the 'perceived self-performance' subscale where the former outscored the latter ($F = 4.06$, $p = .046$, $p\eta^2 = .024$), the two groups of colleagues did not differ significantly ($p >. 05$ in all cases) on the rest of the measures (see Table 1).

Tables 2 to 5 detail the number and proportion of the participating colleagues reporting a positive evaluation of the workshop. An overwhelming proportion of trainees (85.03%) had a positive evaluation of the training content (see Table 2), including recognition of factors that affect teaching (89.76%), promotion of self-reflection (95.81%), appropriateness of the training methods (96.41%), the overall satisfaction with the workshop of oneself (98.80%) and perceived others' satisfaction (86.75%).

Table 1. Means, standard deviations, Cronbach's alphas, and mean of inter-item correlations and the comparison between Senior and Junior Secondary school participants

Subjective Outcome Evaluation (SOE) Scale	Total (N= 171)		Senior (N= 76)		Junior (N= 95)		*F*	*Partial eta-squared*
	M (SD)	*α (Mean#)*	*M (SD)*	*α (Mean#)*	*M (SD)*	*α (Mean#)*		
Training content (16 items)	4.38 (0.41)	.92 (.43)	4.42 (0.44)	.93 (.48)	4.34 (0.38)	.91 (.39)	1.59	0.010
Perceived benefits (9 items)	4.38 (0.43)	.88 (.45)	4.42 (0.46)	.90 (.50)	4.35 (0.40)	.86 (.41)	1.02	0.006
Training quality (5 items)	4.38 (0.45)	.80 (.45)	4.42 (0.46)	.80 (.46)	4.35 (0.44)	.79 (.43)	1.25	0.008
Overall satisfaction (2 items)	4.33 (0.51)	.61 (.45)	4.40 (0.54)	.58 (.43)	4.27 (0.49)	.63 (.47)	2.77	0.017
Instructor quality (5 items)	4.43 (0.42)	.83 (.50)	4.48 (0.44)	.85 (.54)	4.39 (0.40)	.82 (.47)	1.70	0.010
Perceived self-performance (4 items)	4.18 (0.51)	.79 (.49)	4.26 (0.52)	.83 (.56)	4.12 (0.49)	.75 (.43)	4.06*	0.024
Administrative arrangements (6 items)	4.38 (0.45)	.87 (.53)	4.40 (0.47)	.89 (.58)	4.37 (0.43)	.85 (.50)	0.34	0.002
Total scale (31 items)	4.36 (0.37)	.95 (.38)	4.39 (0.40)	.93 (.48)	4.33 (0.34)	.91 (.39)	2.08	0.012

Note. *p <.05 (two-tailed). # Mean inter-item correlations.

Table 2. Summary of the positive views (options 4-5) of the participants towards the content of training

	Perceptions of the training content	N	Agree (4)		Strongly Agree (5)		Positive Response (Options 4-5)		*M*	*SD*
			n	%	*n*	%	*n*	%		
Perceived benefits [a]										
1.	It has strengthened my understanding of the nature of adolescent development.	167	91	53.22	74	44.31	165	98.80	4.43	0.52
2.	It has helped me to cultivate positive attitude to adolescent development.	167	71	42.51	93	55.69	164	98.20	4.54	0.53
3.	It has strengthened my understanding of positive youth development, including its concept, design, and research.	167	85	50.90	77	46.11	162	97.01	4.42	0.59
4.	It has helped me to understand the Tin Ka Ping P.A.T.H.S. Project, including its basic philosophy, design, implementation, and evaluation.	167	82	49.10	79	47.31	161	96.41	4.43	0.59
5.	It has strengthened me to understand the content of the program.	167	86	51.50	74	44.31	160	95.81	4.40	0.57
6.	It has helped me to acquire the attitude, knowledge, and skills that are conducive to the successful implementation of the Tin Ka Ping P.A.T.H.S. Project.	167	89	53.29	59	35.33	148	88.62	4.23	0.66
7.	It has helped me to establish self-help support network and share teaching experiences among the program participants.	166	90	54.22	59	35.54	149	89.76	4.25	0.63

Table 2. (Continued)

Perceptions of the training content		N	Agree (4)		Strongly Agree (5)		Positive Response (Options 4-5)		*M*	*SD*
			n	%	*n*	%	*n*	%		
Perceived benefits [a]										
8.	It has promoted self-reflection.	167	76	45.51	84	50.30	160	95.81	4.46	0.58
9.	It has helped me to recognize factors affecting teaching.	166	83	50.00	66	39.76	149	89.76	4.28	0.68
Training quality [a]										
1.	The training methods and activities are appropriate (e.g., lecture, games, group discussion).	167	77	46.11	84	50.30	161	96.41	4.47	0.57
2.	Training time is appropriate.	166	84	50.60	57	34.34	141	84.94	4.17	0.72
3.	It has met my expectation.	166	80	48.19	63	37.95	143	86.14	4.24	0.68
4.	There was much peer interaction amongst participants.	166	73	43.98	88	53.01	161	96.99	4.50	0.56
5.	Instructor(s) encouraged participants to do the best.	166	71	42.77	91	54.82	162	97.59	4.52	0.55
Overall satisfaction [a]										
1.	Overall speaking, I am satisfied with the training program.	167	82	49.10	83	49.70	165	98.80	4.49	0.52
2.	I think participants are satisfied with the training program.	166	92	55.42	52	31.33	144	86.75	4.17	0.68
Perceptions of the program (whole scale)[a]		167					142*	85.03	4.38	0.41

Note. [a] Scores on the scale/subscale higher than or equal to 4 were treated as positive views.

*Number of participants reporting an overall average score above 4.00.

Table 3. Summary of the positive views (options 4-5) of the participants on the quality of the instructor(s)

Perceptions of the quality of instructor(s)		N	Agree (4)		Strongly Agree (5)		Positive Response (Options 4-5)		*M*	*SD*
			n	%	*n*	%	*n*	%		
1.	The instructor(s) had good mastery of the curriculum.	167	100	59.88	65	38.92	165	98.80	4.38	0.51
2.	The instructor(s) understood the needs of participants.	166	98	59.04	52	31.33	150	90.36	4.22	0.60
3.	The instructor(s) showed good professional attitude.	166	49	29.52	117	70.48	166	100.00	4.70	0.46
4.	The instructor(s)' teaching was clear and easy to understand.	166	86	51.80	67	40.36	153	92.17	4.33	0.62
5.	Overall speaking, I have positive evaluation of the instructor(s)' teaching performance.	167	76	45.51	90	53.89	166	99.40	4.53	0.51
Total scale [a]		167					154*	92.22	4.43	0.42

Note. [a] Scores on the scale higher than or equal to 4 were treated as positive views.

*Number of participants reporting an overall average score above 4.00.

Table 4. Summary of the positive views (options 4-5) of participants towards administrative arrangements

Perceptions of the administrative arrangements		N	Satisfied (4)		Very Satisfied (5)		Positive Response (Options 4-5)		*M*	*SD*
			n	%	*n*	%	*n*	%		
1.	Information obtained before attending the workshop.	171	93	54.39	54	31.58	147	85.96	4.17	0.67
2.	Workshop assigned.	169	101	59.76	58	34.32	159	94.08	4.28	0.57
3.	Location of the workshop.	170	92	54.12	73	42.94	165	97.06	4.40	0.55
4.	Reception provided by training team (e.g., transportation arrangement, refreshments).	170	72	42.35	93	54.71	165	97.06	4.52	0.56
5.	Facilities of the venue.	169	85	50.30	74	43.79	159	94.08	4.38	0.60
6.	Overall speaking, I am satisfied with the administrative arrangements.	171	79	46.20	91	53.22	170	99.42	4.53	0.51
Total scale [a]		171					153*	89.47	4.38	0.45

Note. [a] Scores on the scale higher than or equal to 4 were treated as positive views.

*Number of participants reporting an overall average score above 4.00.

Table 5. Summary of the positive views (options 4-5) of participants towards their own performance in training

	Perceptions of self-performance	N	Agree (4)		Strongly Agree (5)		Positive Response (Options 4-5)		*M*	*SD*
			n	%	*n*	%	*n*	%		
1.	I participated actively in discussion.	171	86	50.29	45	26.32	131	76.61	4.03	0.71
2.	I am willing to apply the specific skills and theories learned from this training program.	171	92	53.80	76	44.44	168	98.25	4.43	0.53
3.	After attending the training program, I have confidence in program implementation.	170	96	56.47	57	33.53	153	90.00	4.23	0.63
4.	Overall speaking, I am satisfied with my performance.	169	93	55.03	42	24.85	135	79.88	4.04	0.68
Total scale [a]		171					122*	71.35	4.18	0.51

Note. [a] Scores on the scale higher than or equal to 4 were treated as positive views.

*Number of participants reporting an overall average score above 4.00.

Table 6. Correlations among the key evaluation components

Variables	1	2	3	4	5	6
1) Training quality (5 items)	-					
2) Perceived benefits (9 items)	0.71***	-				
3) Instructor quality (5 items)	0.64***	0.63***	-			
4) Administrative arrangements (6 items)	0.57***	0.54***	0.65***	-		
5) Self-performance (4 items)	0.55***	0.51***	0.57***	0.56***	-	
6) Overall satisfaction (2 items)	0.74***	0.74***	0.55***	0.54***	0.47***	-

Note. ***p <.001 (two-tailed).

Table 7. Multiple regression analyses predicting perceived benefits and overall satisfaction

Predictors	Perceived Benefits				Overall Satisfaction			
	B	*SE*	*β*	R^2	*B*	*SE*	*β*	R^2
Perceived training quality	0.46	0.07	0.49***	0.57***	0.47	0.08	0.42***	0.65***
Instructor quality	0.23	0.08	0.23***		-0.06	0.09	-0.05	
Administrative arrangements	0.07	0.07	0.07		0.13	0.08	0.11	
Self-performance	0.06	0.06	0.08		-0.01	0.06	-0.01	
Perceived benefits					0.50	0.09	0.42***	

Note. ***p <.001 (two-tailed). B: Unstandardized coefficients; SE: Standard errors; β: Standardized coefficients; R^2: R-squared.

Regarding the perceived quality of instructor(s) (see Table 3), the vast majority of the participants concurred that the instructors had good mastery of the curriculum (98.80%), understood what participants needed (90.36%), were professional throughout (100%), delivered clear and comprehensible teaching (92.17%), and had put on a performance worthy of commendations (99.40%). Additionally, almost all participants (99.42%) felt satisfied with the present administrative arrangements (see Table 4). This particular finding resonates with the data (see Table 4) suggesting that over 90% of participants indicated satisfaction with the workshop's location (97.06%), the facilities of the venue (94.08%), and the reception (97.06%). Furthermore, the majority (79.88%) of trainees expressed satisfaction with their own performance during the training (see Table 5), which is in line with their active participation in discussions (76.61%), willingness to put what they learned into practice (98.25%), and their enhanced confidence to implement a program after attending this workshop (90.00%). Taken together, Hypothesis 1 was supported.

Results of the Pearson's correlational analyses showed that all six sub-scales were all significantly and positively associated with each other (*p*s $<.001$ in all cases, see Table 6). Particularly, the results revealed that participants' overall satisfaction with the training workshop was strongly correlated to the remaining subscales including training quality ($r = 0.74$), perceived benefits of the workshop ($r = 0.74$), instructor quality ($r = 0.55$), administrative arrangements ($r = 0.54$) and self-performance ($r = 0.47$). In short, Hypotheses 2a to 2f were supported.

Two multiple regression analyses were performed with dependent variables being participants' perceived benefits and their overall satisfaction. Regarding perceived benefits, results demonstrated that perceived training quality ($B = 0.46$, SE $= 0.07$, $p <.001$) and instructor quality ($B = 0.23$, SE $= 0.08$, $p <.001$) were significant predictors, supporting Hypotheses 3a and 3b. This model accounted for 56.72% of the variance of participants' perceived benefits (see Table 7). As a follow-up analysis on all the five abovementioned correlates of participants' overall satisfaction ratings, the data showed that only training quality (B = 0.47, SE = 0.08, p <.001) and perceived benefits (B = 0.50, SE = 0.09, p <.001) remained as significant predictors (see Table 7), supporting Hypotheses 4a and 4d. This model accounted for 64.51% of the variance of participants' overall satisfaction ratings.

DISCUSSION

As a means to reinforce positive youth development among youngsters in China in a holistic fashion, the Tin Ka Ping P.A.T.H.S. Project was started in 2011 and has been put into practice in over 30 secondary schools since the academic year 2015-2016. As specified by Shek and colleagues (17, 18), the factor 'people', inclusive of both implementers and participants, is integral to the success of any PYD programs. It is, therefore, imperative that well-designed pre-service training be offered to the potential implementers to assure the smooth delivery of the program (16). Accordingly, similar to previously administered P.A.T.H.S. Project train-the-trainer workshops, we need to address two crucial questions, including 1) how well did the training go and 2) what constituted the key predictor(s) of the trainees' perceived satisfaction and benefits of the current workshop.

Echoing the findings documented in the P.A.T.H.S. Project training evaluation literature, the results were highly supportive of the success of the present training workshop. An overwhelming portion of trainees indicated satisfaction with the workshop in the areas of training content, instructor quality, the administrative arrangements, and their perceived self-performance. Additionally, results of the MANOVA revealed no cross-group (junior vs. senior secondary school colleagues) difference in almost all SOE subscales, suggesting that both groups of trainees had a very positive evaluation of the training program. In short, consistent with previous studies, the trainees held positive views of the different dimensions of the present workshop.

Predictably, results of the correlational analyses confirmed the strong associations amongst the six components (i.e., perceived benefits, self-performance, etc.) of the present training workshop. This again replicated the findings from prior training evaluation studies conducted in both the preparatory year and during the academic year 2015-2016. Specifically, consistent with the hypotheses, measures of trainees' overall satisfaction and perceived benefits were both strongly correlated to one another and to other components such as instructor quality and self-performance.

With regard to predictors of trainees' overall satisfaction and perceived benefits, results of the multiple regression analyses revealed two significant predictors for each outcome measure. Consistent with prior findings and Hypotheses 4a and 4d, both perceived benefits and training quality were significant predictors of the overall satisfaction of the participants. Besides, echoing Hypotheses 3a and 3b, perceived training quality and instructor quality significantly predicted perceived benefits, with training quality being the stronger predictor. Taken together, these findings corroborated the notion that quality of service is key to garnering client satisfaction in a human service program (26).

It is noteworthy that contrary to findings from the preparatory year (see 14), neither administrative arrangements nor self-performance was a significant predictor in the present analyses. This may be attributable to the ceiling effect (i.e., very high satisfaction with the related attributes) and the lack of dispersion for these two variables (22). Alternatively, considering that there were new elements (i.e., lesson demonstrations by selected groups of trainees) for training workshops in the full-implementation phase, and that some attendees were indeed returning participants from the preparatory year workshops, it is conceivable that these participants may be more preoccupied with the training content which was measured by the SOE subscales 'training content' (i.e., the materials) and 'instructor quality' (i.e., the delivery). Nonetheless, at present, we are unable to dismiss any alternative explanations.

It is worth bearing in mind several shortcomings of the current study. First, the predominant reliance on quantitative analyses, in conjunction with the neglect of the open-ended responses, may render the current assessment of colleagues' feedback incomplete. Second, this study only features the subjective evaluation by the prospective implementers. It may be more enlightening to extend the scope of the assessment by also examining how these would-be implementers put their learning into practice (i.e., objective outcome evaluation study on any PYD programs subsequently conducted by the present trainees). Finally, as in other self-report research, social desirability bias may be the genuine reason behind the present supportive findings. People may respond positively with the intent to present themselves in a favorable light (27). However, the self-administered and anonymous nature of the present survey should have disincentivized any social desirability responding tendencies.

In spite of all these limitations, the present study not only underlined the success of the first training workshop in the academic year 2016-2017, but also added to the P.A.T.H.S. Project training evaluation literature by highlighting what dimensions of a train-the-trainer workshop any future trainers should look out for as to maximize participants' perceived benefits and overall satisfaction. As empirical assessments of training programs for implementers in the context of positive youth development programs in China are very rare in the literature, this is a meaningful contribution to the literature.

ACKNOWLEDGMENTS

The preparation for this work and the Tin Ka Ping P.A.T.H.S. Project were financially supported by the Tin Ka Ping Foundation. This chapter is a re-published work based on an article published in the International Journal of Child and Adolescent Health 2018; 11(3) issue.

REFERENCES

[1] Chow GC. Globalization and China's economic development. Pac Econ Rev 2006;11:271-85.

[2] Liang W. China: Globalization and the emergence of a new status quo power? Asian Perspect 2007;31:125-49.

[3] Ng RMK, Li Z. East meets West: Current mental health burdens in Greater China. In: Morgan C, Bhugra D, eds. Principles of social psychiatry, 2nd ed. West Sussex: John Wiley, 2010: 517-30.

[4] Bhat MA, Rather TA. Socio-economic factors and mental health of young people in India and China: An elusive link with globalization. Asian Soc Work Policy Rev 2012;6:1-22.

[5] National Institute of Education Sciences (NIES). Parents' over-emphasis on study puts their children under intense pressure. National Institute of Education Sciences, 2016. URL: http://www.nies.net.cn/zy/wjdc/201603/t20160317_322080.html [Chinese].

[6] Ministry of Education. Guidance by the Ministry of Education on the strengthening of family education. Ministry of Education, 2015. URL: http://www.moe.gov.cn/srcsite/A06/s7053/201510/t20151020_214366.html [Chinese].

[7] Shek DTL, Lee TY, Ma LK. Subjective outcome evaluation of the Tin Ka Ping P.A.T.H.S. Project in China: View of the students. Int Public Health J, in press.

[8] Damon W. What is positive youth development? Ann Am Acad Pol Soc Sci 2004;591:13-24.

[9] Shek DTL, Ma HK, Sun RCF. A brief overview of adolescent developmental problems in Hong Kong. ScientificWorldJournal 2011;11:Article ID 896835. doi:10.1100/2011/896835.

[10] Shek DTL, Sun RCF, eds. Development and evaluation of Positive Adolescent Training through Holistic Social Programs (P.A.T.H.S.). Heidelberg: Springer, 2013.

[11] Shek DTL, Wu FKY. The Project P.A.T.H.S. in Hong Kong: Work done and lessons learned in a decade. J Pediatr Adolesc Gynecol 2016;29:S3-11.

[12] Shek DTL, Han XY. The relationship between subjective outcome evaluation and objective outcome evaluation findings: Evidence from China. Int J Disabil Hum Dev 2014;13:497-503.

[13] Shek DTL, Han XY, Lee TY, Yu L. Subjective outcome evaluation of a positive youth development program in China. Int J Disabil Hum Dev 2014;13:275-83.

[14] Shek DTL, Wu FKY, Leung JTY, Merrick J, eds. Adolescence: Positive youth development programs in Chinese communities. New York: Nova Science, 2016.

[15] Shek DTL, Chung CK, Sun RCF. Positive youth development in mainland China: Evaluation of a training program. In: Shek DTL, Wu FKY, Leung JTY, Merrick J, eds. Adolescence: Positive youth development programs in Chinese communities. New York: Nova Science, 2016:83-95.

[16] Clarke N. The impact of in-service training within social services. Br J Soc Work 2001;31:757-74.

[17] Shek DTL, Sun RCF. The Project P.A.T.H.S. in Hong Kong—lessons learned and implications for positive youth development programs epilogue. ScientificWorldJournal 2012;2012:Article ID 687536. doi: 10.1100/2012/687536.

[18] Wu FKY, Shek DTL. The role of program, people, process, policy and place (5Ps) in the implementation of a positive youth development program. Int J Adolesc Med Health 2012;24:201-6.

[19] Kirkpatrick DL. Evaluating training programs: The four levels. San Francisco, CA: Berrett-Koehler, 1994.

[20] Shek DTL, Leung JTY, Chen M, Chung CK. Evaluation of the training program of a positive youth development program: Tin Ka Ping P.A.T.H.S. project in China. Int Public Health J, in press.

[21] Shek DTL, Lee TY, Wu J. Subjective outcome evaluation of a training program of Tin Ka Ping P.A.T.H.S. Project in China. Int Public Health J, in press.

[22] Shek DTL, Zhu X, Leung JTY. Evaluation of four training programs in mainland China. In: Shek DTL, Wu FKY, Leung JTY, Merrick J, eds. Adolescence: Positive youth development programs in Chinese communities. New York: Nova Science, 2016:111-23.

[23] Shek DTL, Liang RLY, Lee TY. Training program on positive youth development for mainland China. In: Shek DTL, Wu FKY, Leung JTY, Merrick J, eds. Adolescence: Positive youth development programs in Chinese communities. New York: Nova Science, 2016:67-82.

[24] Shek DTL, Chak YLY. Subjective outcome evaluation of the secondary 2 training program of the Project P.A.T.H.S. in Hong Kong. Int J Adolesc Med Health 2011;23:325-32.

[25] Shek DTL, Leung H. Subjective outcome evaluation of the training program of the Project P.A.T.H.S.: Findings based on the revised training program. Int J Disabil Hum Dev 2014;13:267-74.

[26] Larsen DL, Attkisson CC, Hargreaves WA, Nguyen TD. Assessment of client/patient satisfaction: Development of a general scale. Eval Program Plann 1979;2:197-207.

[27] van de Mortel TF. Faking it: Social desirability response bias in self-report research. Aust J Adv Nurs 2008;25:40-8.

Appendix. Content of the first training program of the Tin Ka Ping P.A.T.H.S. project in the academic year 2016-2017 in Jiujiang, China

Junior Group

Day 1 (6.5 hours)	
Themes and objectives	Activities conducted
a) Introduce the latest progress of the Tin Ka Ping P.A.T.H.S. Project during the full implementation phase (2016-2017); b) Familiarize the attendees with teaching units relevant to the constructs "Social Competence" (SC) and "Prosocial Norms" (PN) c) Provide opportunities for school delegates to share their experience on how to deliver certain teaching units.	1) *Introduce the Tin Ka Ping P.A.T.H.S. Project and the professional team, ice-breaking and warm-up activities; 2) *Introduce the schedule and arrangement of the Train-the-trainer program; 3) *Provide updates on the Tin Ka Ping P.A.T.H.S. Project website; 4) *Report the implementation of the Co-Walker Scheme; 5) *Report the results of evaluation of the third training program (in the academic year 2015-2016) in Changchun; 6) Lecture on the constructs of "Social Competence" (SC) and "Prosocial Norms" (PN) and the content of units designed based on these two constructs and; 7) Interactive lecture on the unit BO (Bonding) 2.2, followed by experience sharing and Question and Answer (Q&A) sessions; 8) Interactive lecture on the unit SD (Self-determination) 1.1, followed by experience sharing and Q&A sessions; 9) Interactive lecture on the unit EC (Emotional competence) 2.3, followed by experience sharing and Q&A sessions.

Note. *Activities conducted together with the Senior Group.

(Continued)

Day 2 (7.5 hours)	
Themes and objectives	Activities conducted
a) Provide opportunities for representatives from Jiujiang and other participating institutions to share their teaching experiences and offer pointers on how to properly deliver the lessons; b) Familiarize the trainees with the teaching techniques of the Tin Ka Ping P.A.T.H.S. Project teaching units.	1) *Warm-up activities and; 2) *Lesson demonstrations by four experienced teachers from the four participating schools plus a Q&A session for each demonstration session.
Day 3 (3 hours)	
Themes and objectives	Activities conducted
a) Familiarize the colleagues with the constructs and teaching units; b) Familiarize the trainees with the teaching techniques of the Tin Ka Ping P.A.T.H.S. Project teaching units; c) Familiarize the participants with the teaching units related to the construct of "Prosocial Norms" (PN).	1) Warm-up activities; 2) Lecture on the constructs of "Prosocial Norms" (PN) and the contents of the unit; 3) Sharing and discussion sessions by the participating schools; 4) *Introduction of the findings of course evaluation in the academic year 2015-2016; 5) *Wrapping up and self-reflection; and 6) *Conclusion and final remarks.

Note. *Activities conducted together with the Senior Group.

Senior Group

Day 1 (6.5 hours)	
Themes and objectives	Activities conducted
a) Introduce the latest progress of the Tin Ka Ping P.A.T.H.S. Project during the full implementation phase (2016-2017); b) Familiarize the attendees with the constructs and teaching units.	1) *Introduce the Tin Ka Ping P.A.T.H.S. Project and the professional team, ice-breaking and warm-up activities; 2) *Introduce the schedule and arrangement of the Train-the-trainer program;

Note. *Activities conducted together with the Junior Group.

(Continued)

Senior Group

Day 1 (6.5 hours)	
Themes and objectives	Activities conducted
	3) *Provide updates on the Tin Ka Ping P.A.T.H.S. Project website; 4) *Report the implementation of the Co-Walker Scheme; 5) *Report the results of evaluation of the third training program (in the academic year 2015-2016) in Changchun; 6) Lecture on the constructs of "Behavioral Competence" (BC) and "Self-efficacy" (SE) and the content of teaching units designed based on these two constructs; 7) Lecture on the constructs of "Clear and Positive Identity" (ID) and "Self-efficacy" (SE) and the content of teaching units designed based on these two constructs; 8) Lecture on the constructs of "Social Competence" (SC) and "Clear and Positive Identity" (ID) and the content of teaching units designed based on these two constructs; 9) Sharing session from participating schools; 10) Group discussion and Q&A session.

Note. *Activities conducted together with the Junior Group.

(Continued)

Day 2 (7.5 hours)	
Themes and objectives	Activities conducted
a) Provide opportunities for representatives from Jiujiang and other participating institutions to share their teaching experiences and offer pointers on how to properly deliver the lessons; b) Familiarize the trainees with the teaching techniques of the Tin Ka Ping P.A.T.H.S. Project teaching units.	1) *Warm-up activities and; 2) *Lesson demonstrations by four experienced teachers from the four participating schools plus a Q&A session for each demonstration session.
Day 3 (3 hours)	
Themes and objectives	Activities conducted
a) Familiarize the colleagues with the constructs and teaching units; b) Familiarize the trainees with the teaching techniques of the Tin Ka Ping P.A.T.H.S. Project teaching units; c) Familiarize the participants with the teaching units related to the constructs of "Bonding" (BO), "Resilience" (RE) and "Emotional Competence" (EC).	1) Warm-up activities; 2) Lecture on the constructs of "Bonding" (BO), "Resilience" (RE) and "Emotional Competence" (EC) and the contents of the teaching units designed based on these three constructs; 3) Sharing and discussion sessions by the participating schools; 4) *Introduction of the findings of course evaluation in the academic year 2015-2016; 5) *Wrapping up and self-reflection; and 6) *Conclusion and final remarks.

Note. * Activities conducted together with the Junior Group.

In: Childhood and Adolescence
Editor: Joav Merrick
ISBN: 978-1-53613-574-9

Chapter 6

A QUALITATIVE STUDY ON THE ROLE OF GENDER IN THE HEALTH AND DEVELOPMENT OF ADOLESCENTS IN DISADVANTAGED COMMUNITIES IN IBADAN, NIGERIA

Adesola O Olumide**, MBBS, MPH, FWACP, FMCPH and Oladosu A Ojengbede, BSc, MBBS, FMCOG, FWACS, FICS

Institute of Child Health and Department of Obstetrics and Gynaecology, University of Ibadan and University College Hospital, Ibadan, Nigeria

This study explored gender influences on the health and development of adolescents residing in disadvantaged communities in Ibadan, Nigeria. Findings are from the Ibadan (Nigeria) site of the multi-city Wellbeing of Adolescents in Vulnerable Environments (WAVE) study. A total of 132 respondents comprising 20 adult key informants and 112 adolescents (20 in-depth interviewees, 11 photovoice participants and 81 participants in

* Correspondence: Adesola O Olumide, University of Ibadan and University College Hospital, 200001 Ibadan, Nigeria. Email: daisyolu@yahoo.co.uk; aoolumide@com.ui.edu.ng.

eight community mapping and FGDs) participated. Findings revealed that gender influenced everyday activities, health and social life of the adolescents. Females generally performed more chores than the males. Younger adolescent males also performed a range of chores although the older adolescent males did considerably fewer chores. Males were not favoured over females with respect to accessing education or healthcare. The study highlighted that male adolescents were sometimes favoured over the females. Interventions to reduce gender inequities could be useful in ensuring healthy development of adolescents in the study area.

INTRODUCTION

Adolescents are individuals aged 10-19 years old and they are undergoing physical, mental and psychological changes which are characteristic of the transition from childhood to adulthood (1, 2). Adolescents constitute approximately a fifth of the world population (3) and they are generally viewed as healthy. They however contribute to the global burden of disease and injury (4, 5) and their tendency to experiment and initiate health-risk behaviours pose additional risks to their health and development (2, 3). Gore et al. (4) in their review of the Global Burden of Disease (GBD), injuries and risk factors in young people reported that neuropsychiatric disorders, unintentional injuries, and infectious and parasitic diseases were the most common causes of years of life lost due to disabilities among this population. An important finding from that review was the fact that across regions, girls aged 15 to 19 years had significantly higher disability-adjusted life year (DALY) rates compared to their male counterparts (4).

Over the years, gender has been identified as a factor influencing health and development (6-8). Burnette (9) described gender as, "the social behaviours, lifestyle, and personality characteristics that women and men are expected to exhibit" (9). Existing literature reveal that male and female gender roles are passed on through socialization within the family, school, community and society at large (6, 10, 11). For instance, male adolescents are taught to be assertive and to be the breadwinners while females are taught to be meek and submissive (6, 12). The socialization of gender often commences early, with girls and boys being treated differently from the time they are born (6). Although this differential treatment is sometimes harmless, situations exist in which they become discriminatory and place a limitation on the attainment of individual and collective goals (13). Previous studies and observations reveal that the different gender roles and expectations are learnt from birth, however, these differences often become pronounced as children attain puberty and transit to adulthood (14, 15). For example, restriction of the movement of females within the neighbourhood often commence about the time that children attain puberty. This movement restriction is often attributed to the need to "protect" the females from sexual and other types of harm (7, 15). A review of the literature to understand factors that shape gender attitudes in early adolescence by Kågesten et al. (2016) revealed that young adolescents in different settings support existing gender-biased norms and that parents and other adults within the society play major roles in entrenching these beliefs (7).

Gender disparities have implications for the health and development of adolescents—especially adolescent girls, because these disparities often favour the boys unduly (16, 17). Some studies have however demonstrated that some gender-based norms such as those that define men as being invincible could affect men adversely in terms of reducing the tendency for men to seek help when they require it. Many of these norms are also introduced early in life (12, 18). Fatusi and Hindin (19), posited that in developing countries, gender has a significant influence on various aspects of adolescent health and development including mobility, access to health services, and youth engagement (19). In Nigeria, as in many developing countries, gender plays an important role in virtually all facets of life (10, 20, 21).

Researchers have described the association between gender and various health behaviours, outcomes, and help-seeking behaviours (18, 19, 22). Findings from these studies indicate that a person's gender might preclude access to health or other services (12, 15). Issues relating to such gender-based discrimination have thus received attention globally and locally. Interventions including legislation and female-centred programmes have been developed in an attempt to improve the lot of the female child/

adolescent who is often at the receiving end of discriminatory gender norms (13, 23). Many of these programmes have been in place for decades and it is expected that in contemporary times, gender inequities should have been eliminated or at least reduced as a result of implementation of these interventions. A literature search revealed a gap in current knowledge on the influence of gender on adolescent health and development in Nigeria, a rapidly developing country. Such information is required to guide the development of relevant adolescent-centred interventions not only in Nigeria, but in other countries that have a considerable population of adolescents and young people. The aim of this study was thus to explore the ways in which gender influenced the lived experiences of adolescents residing in disadvantaged communities within Ibadan. We focused on adolescents residing in disadvantaged environments because they are often marginalized, have limited access to health and other facilities and the influence of gender on everyday activities is often pronounced in poorer communities and nations (21, 24). Our study findings will (i) contribute to existing knowledge on the influence of gender norms in adolescent health and development and (ii) highlight possible aspects of gender norms that might require urgent interventions in order to eliminate gender inequity and promote an environment which encourages maximal healthy growth and development of both male and female adolescents.

OUR STUDY

Data for this paper were from a multi-city study conducted in the following five global cities: Baltimore, United States; Delhi, India; Ibadan, Nigeria; Johannesburg, South Africa; and Shanghai, China. The study was conducted in two phases—the first phase employed a qualitative research approach, whereas the second phase utilized a quantitative research approach. Findings presented here are based on the qualitative results from the Ibadan site only. The same methods were utilized for data collection in all the study sites (25-27).

In Ibadan, the adolescents were selected from disadvantaged neighbourhoods in one (Ibadan North) of the five Local Government Areas that constitute Ibadan municipality. These neighbourhoods were purposively selected after expert interviews with the Medical Officer of Health and other professionals working with adolescents in Ibadan North Local Government Area. The selected neighbourhoods are known to be disadvantaged in terms of having a large number of overcrowded housing, inadequate social amenities and high school dropout rates compared with better-off locations within the Local Government Area. Data were collected through a variety of approaches including key informant interviews, in-depth interviews, community mapping, Focus Group Discussion (FGD) and photovoice exercises. Twenty key informants were purposively selected in order to ensure a broad range of adults who were knowledgeable about adolescent issues and who worked with adolescents in various capacities within the study area participated. The key informants comprised secondary school teachers, health workers, and heads or staff of adolescent-centred organizations located within the Ibadan North Local Government Area (LGA). In-depth interviews, community mapping, FGDs and photovoice sessions were conducted among adolescents aged 15 to 19 years. Adolescent recruitment was facilitated by the key informants and other adults within the LGA.

The sample size for the study was 132 comprising of 20 key informants and 112 adolescents aged 15 to 19 years. The 112 adolescents included 20 in-depth interviewees, 81 adolescents who participated in 10 community mapping and FGD sessions, and 11 adolescents who participated in the photovoice activity. Appropriate interview guides were developed for all the data collection methods and, in Ibadan, these instruments were translated from English to Yoruba, the predominant language in the study area and back translated (28) to ensure that the original meanings were retained. The key informant interviews and in-depth interviews each lasted approximately 45 minutes to more than an hour. The community mapping and FGDs were day-long activities. Each of the ten community mapping and FGD sessions comprised eight adolescent participants (although in one group, there were nine adolescents). There were four CM and FGDs groups each for male and female and younger (15-17 years) and older (18 and to 19 years) adolescents. The adolescents first participated in the community mapping exercise during which they drew a map of their community and located selected places on the maps. Following this, they participated in the FGDs where additional questions on adolescent health and development were discussed. The photovoice activities included training and debriefing/ discussion sessions and were conducted over about ten days. The photovoice exercise was facilitated by research staff who were experienced in conducting research and in photography. They guided the adolescents through the basics of photography and also explained the use of photographs for capturing health messages. Each day, the adolescents participating in the photovoice sessions reported to the study office where they were given a brief talk on photovoice; they then went into the community to take pictures that reflected what they understood by health. At the end of the day, all the adolescents returned to the study office where the pictures were discussed with one of the investigators and the photovoice consultants. At the end of the photovoice exercise, each adolescent selected a maximum of 10 pictures that they believed represented their top 10 pictures and they provided captions for each of the pictures. The photovoice discussions were recorded digitally. [Details of the photovoice methods have been reported in a previous publication (29)]. Each adolescent participated in only one of the different methods used.

The process of qualitative data analysis for the entire study was led by the lead qualitative researcher from Baltimore in order to ensure consistency across all the study sites. Details of this process have been described in previous publications (25, 26). In each study site, one of the site investigators took the lead in the analysis (AO coordinated the qualitative data analysis at the Ibadan site). All interviews were recorded digitally, translated and then transcribed verbatim. The typed transcripts were analyzed using ATLAS.ti software (Scientific Software, Berlin; version 7.5.10) (30). The initial code development was coordinated by the overall lead qualitative investigator, with input from the investigators in all the sites. In Ibadan, two teams (each comprising two research staff) coded each transcript. All the codes were discussed and where there were discrepancies, the coders and the investigator discussed these discrepancies and agreed on the final code(s) to be used. For the current paper, the qualitative data were analyzed using a constant comparison approach (31, 32). The investigators read through the previously coded transcripts and identified segments of the transcripts relevant to the current paper that required additional codes or sub-codes. Additional codes were created and applied as required. After coding was completed, the codes were categorized into broader themes. Matrices of relevant themes were then run to explore relationships between themes and the different categories of respondents.

Trustworthiness of the data

Measures were taken to ensure trustworthiness of our data in line with guidelines described by Shenton (33). These measures included having a clear plan for data collection and analysis, discussion of all codes with coding teams, clarification of statements with the interviewers and presentation of findings to colleagues knowledgeable in this field. Ethical approval was obtained from the Committee on Human Research at the Johns Hopkins University (the coordinating institution for the study) and from the Ethics committees of all the collaborating institutions. In Ibadan, approval was also obtained from the University of Ibadan/University College Hospital, Ibadan, Ethical Review Committee. Adults and adolescents aged 18 and 19 years and parents/guardians of adolescents aged 15 to 17 years provided written informed consent and the adolescents aged 15 to 17 years also provided informed assent. For a few adolescents aged 15 to 17 years who were matured minors, all efforts were undertaken by the investigators to ensure that they were indeed mature minors and were able to provide consent, and they were then taken through the process of informed consent.

FINDINGS

The socio-demographic characteristics of the study participants are presented in Table 1. The key informants comprised secondary school teachers and other adults working with adolescents in non-governmental organizations and religious organizations. There were 112 adolescents aged 15 to 19 years.

Table 1. Characteristics of study participants

Participant category		N	%
Key Informants (*n* = 20)	Male	8	40.0
	Female	12	60.0
In-depth interviewees (*n* = 20)			
Gender	Male	10	50.0
	Female	10	50.0
Age group	15 – 17	10	50.0
	18 – 19	10	50.0
Community mapping and FGD(*n* = 81)			
Gender	Male	41	50.6
	Female	40	49.4
Age group	15 – 17	40	49.4
	18 – 19	41	50.6
Photovoice (*n* = 11)			
Gender	Male	5	45.5
	Female	6	54.5
Age group	15 – 17	6	54.5
	18 – 19	5	45.5

The following themes based on the role of gender in adolescent health and development were developed: (a) Gender and everyday experiences, (b) Gender and health/disease, (c) Gender and social life, and (d) Gender and aspirations. Each of these themes is discussed in the subsequent sections.

Theme 1: Gender and everyday experiences

The participants provided information on the role of gender in everyday experiences. These covered a number of areas including gender roles at the household level, and schooling or work experiences.

Household experiences: Generally, the participants reported that gender influenced adolescents' experiences at the household level and this was evident in the type and amount of household chores that adolescents were required to undertake. Both males and females performed domestic chores, although females did more chores and there were differences in the types of chores that the males and females performed. The females often cooked, took care of the house and fetched water. A common chore performed by the males was fetching water. A 15-year-old male adolescent in describing the gender differences in everyday life remarked, "The major difference is that the girls do more work than the boys."

The following conversion ensued between a 19 year old female and the interviewer:

> Interviewer: What is the difference between challenges that male and female youth face?
>
> Respondent: Males do not want to do domestic work; it is the females that do it
>
> Interviewer: What types of domestic work?
>
> Respondent: Like cooking, washing and fetching water, though males also do it but it is the females that do it most of the time

A notable finding that emerged was that whereas the younger adolescent males (15-16 years old) who were still schooling mentioned undertaking various household chores, younger adolescent males who were employed (full-time or as apprentices) and the older adolescent males rarely performed any household chores (This difference can be seen in the narratives below).

A 16 year old male adolescent who was still enrolled in school described his typical week thus:

> Every morning when I wake up, I do my household chores: wash plates and cloths, sweep, fetch water, etc. and then go to school. I always go to the shop immediately I return from school by 2:00pm and I return home when it is 7:45pm in the evening.

He also performed a number of chores during the weekend. He further explained:

> Saturday is the day I do my household chores: I wash my clothes, do environmental sanitation [clean the surroundings of my house] and attend Quranic School. I am always at home on Sundays doing household chores: wash plates and cloths, sweep, fetch water, etc. and later in the day visit my friends.

An 18 year old male adolescent who was no longer enrolled in school in describing his typical week stated, 'During the week, I go to my friends, play with my friends and go back home … I go out to church come back … go to other places. That's it'. His typical week-end was spent doing the following, 'Sometimes on weekends … I go out, sometimes I go to the market to buy some things. Sometimes I go out with my friends and then come back home to rest'.

It thus appears that as the males grew older and attained some level of independence they stopped performing household chores. On the contrary, the females still performed household chores irrespective of age or employment status.

An excerpt of the interview conducted with one of the female respondents (a 15 year old; student and part-time apprentice) is below:

> Respondent: The females do household chores and the males go to their work/office
>
> Interviewer: What types of household chores do the females do at home?
>
> Respondent: … like washing clothes, washing plates, fetching water and cooking and taking care of the children
>
> Interviewer: What about males?
>
> Respondent: They go to work

Interviewer: What types of work?

Respondent: Like office work and some are involved in personal business

Interviewer: Is it all of them (the males)?

Respondent: Yes

Interviewer: Don't the males do any household chores?

Respondent: No

Some females mentioned being overburdened by these chores. For instance, a 15 year old female who was still schooling and also a part-time apprentice when asked about the differences in challenges faced by male and female youth in her community stated, 'Females are encumbered with household chores, ……..'

Schooling or work experiences: The participants did not mention any gender differences in schooling/ work. They opined that male and females were equally expected to attend school and they did attend school, whereas apprentices or those working went to work on week days. The adolescents remarked that there was limited time for relaxation during the week. In addition, students sometimes had to attend additional lessons in school on Saturdays, whereas apprentices had to go to work on Saturdays. Christians usually attended church services on Sundays.

Theme 2: Gender and health or disease

A number of disease and health-related issues affecting male and female adolescents were mentioned by the adolescents and key informants. Sub-themes related to health and disease that were discussed included reproductive health issues, violence and substance abuse and other general problems such as water-borne diseases, malaria and mental health problems.

Reproductive health issues: The females were generally perceived to be more affected by sexual and reproductive health problems. Some reasons for this were that females were not as strong "physically" as the boys and thus were vulnerable to sexual and other forms of harassment. In addition, girls could get pregnant and when this occurred, they experienced the consequences of unplanned pregnancy such as, abortions complications, and school dropout. A key informant stated:

> … like I've said before, boys don't suffer from abortion, they don't suffer from unwanted pregnancies, but they can suffer from STIs, they can suffer from HIV/ AIDS, even though not as fast as the females, but they also suffer from it (Key Informant, Medical Officer of Health).

Females were also described as being more vulnerable to unwanted sexual solicitations that might result in violence if they did not want to date the young men who wanted to date them. The following conversation ensued between one of the 18 year old male in-depth interviewees and a research interviewer:

> Interviewer: the boys and girls that are living in that community and are they facing any challenges?
>
> Respondent: The challenges they are facing is that girls may go out, and while walking from one street to another, some boys may attack them and may rape them … do whatever with them. That's it.

Gender, substance use and safety/violence: The participants reported that male adolescents were more likely to use illicit drugs than were the females. When describing the challenges males within her community encounter, a 16 year old female adolescent said, '… … they [the males] too roam about the street without anything to do and smoke marijuana'.

The study participants associated the use of these substances with the occurrence of violence within the community. The interviewees also mentioned that males and females could be victims of violence; however, females were more at risk. Boys and men were more likely to be perpetrators of violence and fights sometimes broke out when the young men were gambling or if they had been drinking alcohol. Participants mentioned that females were often advised to keep away from some places within the neighbourhood in order to avoid being attacked by hoodlums. Some places within the Local Government Area were notorious as hangout spots for drug addicts who were responsible for spates of violence that often required in intervention by the police.

Another health issue discussed was the perception of safety and behaviours regarding safety, and perpetration of violence within the community. On the whole, most respondents felt safe within most parts of the community during the day. However, males could move around easily but females could not do so, especially at nights, because of safety concerns. According to a 17 year old male in-depth interviewee, '… it is not safe for girls to go out in the night in this community. So, their parents do not allow them to go out at night.' A 15-year-old respondent buttressed this by concluding, 'boys move around more 'freely'.

Mental health problems were considered to be uncommon—although when mentioned, the participants stated that mental health problems were a consequence of psychoactive substance abuse.

Gender and access to healthcare: The male and female adolescents generally had similar knowledge about where to access good health care and, on the whole, there were no striking gender-related barriers to accessing healthcare. Male and female adolescents readily identified sources of healthcare within the study area and they located these on the community maps that they drew.

The adult key informants noted that, generally, adolescents as a group did not have ready access to health services. A female key informant remarked:

> I believe that, especially [with regards to] reproductive health services, we are failing…or we have fallen short; because …. we don't have enough avenues open to these children, inviting [attractive] enough for them to walk in and ask questions or be educated and prevent some of these outcomes that we eventually see in them.

A general barrier to accessing these services mentioned by the adolescents and key informants was the cost of healthcare services. This barrier was not restricted to either males or females. In addition, the participants noted that parents usually determined the facilities where adolescents obtained health care and this often depended on their parents' knowledge of where to obtain health care and what the parents could afford.

The participants explained that adolescents seldom sought for health information from the Internet. All categories of participants – male and female adolescents and the key informants were unanimous in their assertion that males were more versatile in the use of the internet in general and sourced for information from the Internet more frequently than the females.

Theme 3: Gender and social life

Gender had a significant influence on the social life of the adolescents within the study area. Male adolescents were perceived to move around within the neighbourhood freely compared to the females although this was not viewed as a disadvantage. Most respondents felt that it was important to restrict the movement of females who were more vulnerable physically compared to the males. The male adolescents were more knowledgeable than females about recreation centres and places where youth could gather to relax and readily located them on the community maps.

There were differences in the leisure activities undertaken by the male and female adolescents. The findings revealed that females often stayed at home and watched films or visited friends and spent the time chatting with their friends. A 15- year old female mentioned, "I go to a friend's place to 'gist' before I go to my partner's place."

A 19 year old female adolescent asserted,

> … I don't go anywhere. I stay at home to read my books, to do house work and to do all necessary things which I need to do at home. … … I don't do anything as fun…. maybe sometimes I go out with my friend and my sister.

The males were more involved in outdoor activities such as sport (they played football in playing grounds within the neighbourhood). In addition, boys frequently visited friends, utilized cybercafés, went to night clubs and public viewing centres where they watched football matches etc. A16 year old male adolescent stated,

> During the weekend - I am only free on Sunday, I go to work on Saturdays, but on Sunday after coming back from church, I go to the field to play ball, after I finish playing ball, I go home to have my bath and I have my rest that is all.

Males and females also participated actively in religious activities. A common leisure activity undertaken by the males and females over the weekend was attending activities – choir practice in church. One of the female adolescents remarked, 'The way I spend my weekend...... in the morning, I wash clothes and I go to choir practice when it is 4:00pm'. In addition, some of the females mentioned that there was a faith-based girls' club within their community where girls were taught about various health issues. None of the participants mentioned a similar club that targeted boys.

An 18-year-old male reported that with respect to mental health and wellbeing, males were at an advantage compared to the females because the males could engage in extra-curricular activities when they were worried to get over their problems but that girls could not do this. He stated:

> What we, the male are facing is different from what female are facing because if we are not happy we can go to play ball or table tennis to wipe away the sorrow but they don't have this opportunity.

Theme 4: Gender and aspirations

Male and female adolescents aspired to be the best in their endeavours, although females' aspirations were more likely to be adversely affected if they became pregnant. The male adolescents appeared to be under some pressure to attain their goals so that they could, 'take care of their girlfriends and eventually wives'. One of the 18-year-old male adolescents stated:

> The females focus on their own lives for the future; but the males face the problem of how to get their daily bread and how things would work out well for them [i.e., how they will make progress in life] before they want to date any girl.

DISCUSSION

The study findings confirm that gender plays an important role in adolescent health and development including everyday experiences, health, social life and their aspirations. On the whole, these findings reflect the patriarchal nature of the study area (communities within Ibadan North, Nigeria) in which males are often at an advantage compared to females and this is also typical of many societies within and outside of Africa (6, 8, 10, 34).

Findings on gender and everyday experiences were largely consistent with previous literature and somewhat skewed in favour of the males. However, a notable difference was that the younger adolescent males performed several chores, although the males appeared to do less as they grew older. Females were involved in cooking, cleaning and various other chores within the home while the males often fetched water and cleaned the household surroundings. This is in line with the mothering/ child caring roles generally expected of females while men who are viewed as physically stronger are expected to carry out the more physically demanding tasks (6, 8). The volume of chores undertaken was tilted in favour of the males as they generally did less than the females. This is similar to what has been reported in older and contemporary literature (6, 8, 10, 17, 20, 21, 34). A recent UNICEF report (17) and other literature have revealed that as early as childhood, girls spend considerably more hours performing household chores than boys and this disparity persists to adolescence (16). Although, taking part in household chores is part of healthy growth and development, the gender discrepancy in performance of household chores could have negative effects on females. First, being overburdened with chores means that compared to the males, females have limited time to engage in other leisure activities such as interacting with their peers and playing; these are activities that are essential for healthy development. Furthermore, females could be socialized into thinking that performing household chores are the only roles they can fulfil and may not aspire to attain other dreams. In many societies, females are brought up believing these are the only roles they are to play because they are being prepared to become future wives (35). Although there have been efforts to bridge the inequity between males and females (13, 23), more interventions are still required to provide females with a supportive environment to enable them acquire other skills in the same way as their male counterparts.

The schooling and work experiences of the males and females were generally similar. Both males and females attended school or went to their places of work during the week and had some time off over the weekends. This is quite contrary to many reports that show that fewer numbers of females especially those residing in poorer communities and in developing countries attend school compared to their male counterparts (16). Data from the 2015 UNESCO Education For All (EFA) report indicated that in many countries the disparities in male-female attendance in school had reduced although the situation was still less than optimal, especially among students in secondary schools (36). The absence of a perceived difference in access to education among males and females expressed by all our participants could be because the study was conducted in South Western Nigeria. Anecdotally, people in the South-Western part of the country have embraced education; parents are generally in favour of education for both male and female children, and age-long gender inequalities in education are gradually being eroded. The 2013 National Demographic and Health Survey (NDHS) data revealed that Net Attendance Ratio (NAR) for secondary school, (which is the percentage of the secondary school population attending secondary school) for males and females aged 13 to 18 years in Oyo state, South Western Nigeria were 58.1% and 68.5% respectively with a Gender Parity Index (the ratio of the secondary school NAR for females to the NAR for males) of 1.18 compared to a GPI of 0.86 nationally (37). Our findings on access to educational and aspirations are thus a welcome development and additional efforts need to be put in place to sustain access to education among both males and females in the study area.

The main categories of health problems emphasized were Sexual and Reproductive Health (SRH), substance use and safety/violence. Findings were similar to other studies and underscored the higher vulnerability of females to SRH problems and violence. Other literature have similarly highlighted the vulnerability of females to sexual coercion and violence and the consequences of unplanned pregnancy (38, 39). Males also engage in unsafe sex, however, the fact that males "do not get pregnant," as emphasized by one of our participants makes girls at risk of more consequences of unsafe sex. Parents and guardians thus place restrictions on mobility of females in an attempt to protect them from the consequences of unsafe sex. This is in line with existing literature which reveal that parents and guardians often limit the movement of girls (especially those residing in low and middle income countries) within the community when they attain puberty, because of the fear of male attention, sexual solicitations and sexual violence (6, 24, 40). This was confirmed by our participants as they expressed that mobility was often restricted for girls because of concerns for their safety. With respect to problems of violence and psychoactive substance use, males were stated to be more likely to be perpetrators of violence and to use psychoactive substances. This has also been reported by other researchers (24, 39).

Key informants expressed concern that there were limited facilities within the community that were adolescent-friendly and that this reduced the options of care available to both males and females. The adolescents did not express any difference in access to health care for males or females. This was probably because many of the adolescents were residing with their parents or guardians who were largely responsible for the choice and type of healthcare utilized. Cost of services was mentioned as a barrier to accessing healthcare by both males and females. This issue needs to be addressed to promote adolescent health and well-being within the study area.

In the current study, the social life of the females compared to the males was restricted. On the other hand, the male adolescents were free to go out within and outside the community and participate in various activity-oriented games. Other researchers have similarly reported that females experience more restrictions in mobility within their neighbourhoods compared with men who are allowed to move freely and engage in various leisure activities within the community (7, 24). The females might thus be laying the foundation for a future sedentary lifestyle which would become a problem in the future. This finding highlights a need for interventions to encourage girls to be involved in extracurricular activities within the study area. This is in line with the WHO recommendation that advocates that children aged 5-17 years require at least an hour of daily physical activity (24). To facilitate this, government and adolescent-focused non-governmental organizations need to provide safe places for girls within the community where they can visit and engage in various sports and exercises. Interventions that encourage adolescent males to continue to participate in sporting activities are also necessary to sustain their current levels of activity.

It is worthy of note that in this study, the male and female adolescents equally aspired to attain their personal goals. There was however additional pressure on the young men to become achievers because they would have to 'take care of their future families'. While this might be the society's way of training men to take charge and prepare them for the role of family head in future, it could also place undue pressure on them and set the stage for stress which could progress to becoming a risk for development of non-Communicable diseases in the future. This expectation of men is not peculiar to our environment as society generally ascribes the role of provider to them (6) and men in turn view this as a part of their masculinity (41).

Conclusion

The study findings are comparable with existing literature confirming that (i) differences in gender roles and expectations of male and female adolescents are still present in our society and (ii) males are still at an advantage compared to their female counterparts. In spite of this, a laudable finding was the absence of gender discrimination in perceived access to education and healthcare.

In view of the study findings, the following recommendations are made:

- Government and parents should sustain the progress made in reducing the gender disparities in access to education and health care by ensuring that boys and girls continue to have access to these basic amenities. However, measures to reduce the cost of healthcare for all adolescents need to be instituted.
- Parents and guardians should encourage older adolescent males to participate in household chores in order not to overburden the females and to ensure a balance in development for both males and females.
- Governments and community leaders should provide and ensure safe spaces within the community where females can interact and participate in extracurricular activities.
- Parents and others in the society should strike a balance when bringing up males so that they do not feel unduly pressured about their future roles as providers. Interventions which ensure that females access good quality education and are gainfully employed is one way of reducing the burden of "provider" on the males.

In spite of the robust information obtained in this study the qualitative design that was utilized limits over-generalization of the study findings beyond the participants and the study area. An important strength of this study however, was the use of various methods of data collection which ensured in-depth information was obtained and facilitated triangulation of the findings across the different categories of respondents The findings therefore add to existing knowledge on the influence of gender on adolescent health and development and highlight the need for more pro-active interventions to address and hopefully eliminate detrimental aspects of gender roles and expectations on males and females in our study area and in many similar societies.

ACKNOWLEDGMENTS

Authors' contributions. – AOO and OAO were the investigators for the WAVE study in Ibadan and were involved in all the aspects of the study. Both investigators were involved in the write up of the current manuscript and approved the final manuscript.

The WAVE study was funded in Ibadan by The Bill and Melinda Gates Institute at Johns Hopkins Bloomberg School of Public Health through its funding to The Centre for Population and Reproductive Health (JHSPH no. 2000075627), University of Ibadan. In the other sites, the WAVE study was funded by The Young Health Program, a partnership between AstraZeneca, Johns Hopkins Bloomberg School of Public Health and Plan International.

The authors acknowledge Prof A. J. Onwuegbuzie for assistance with proof-reading and editing the manuscript, Mr. E. Adebayo and Ms. A. Adewale for assistance with proof-reading the final manuscript. The authors also acknowledge all the research staff and the study participants.

The authors have no known conflicts of interest.

REFERENCES

[1] Cherry AL, Baltag V, Dillon ME. International handbook on adolescent health and development: The public health response. Cham: Springer, 2016.

[2] McNeely C, Blanchard J. The teen years explained: A guide to healthy adolescent development. Baltimore, MD: Center Adolescent Health, Johns Hopkins Bloomberg School of Public Health, 2009.

[3] UNICEF. Progress for Children. A report card on adolescents. Geneva: UNICEF, 2012.

[4] Gore F, Bloem P, Patton GC, Ferguson J, Joseph V, Coffey C, et al. Global burden of disease in young people aged 10-24 years: A systematic analysis. Lancet 2011;377(9783):2093-102.

[5] Mokdad AH, Forouzanfar MH, Daoud F, Mokdad AA, El Bcheraoui C, Moradi-Lakeh M, et al. Global burden of diseases, injuries, and risk factors for young people's health during 1990–2013: A systematic analysis for the Global Burden of Disease Study 2013. Lancet 2016;387:2383-401.

[6] Holmes M. Gender and everyday life. New York: Routledge, 2009.

[7] Kågesten A, Gibbs S, Blum RW, Moreau C, Chandra-Mouli V, Herbert A, et al. Understanding Factors that Shape Gender Attitudes in Early Adolescence Globally: A Mixed-Methods Systematic Review. PLoS One 2016;11(6):e0157805.

[8] Silberschmidt M. Women forget that men are the masters: Gender antagonism and socio-economic change in Kisii District, Kenya: Nordic Africa Institute, 1999.

[9] Burnette MM. Gender, gender identity and sexuality. In: McAnulty RD, Burnette MM, eds. Sex and sexuality, Sexuality today: trends and controversies. Westport, CT: Praeger, 2006:185-201.

[10] Akpotor J. Patriarchy and emergent gender equality in Nigeria. Int J Res 2016;3(12):230-48.

[11] Ryle R. Questioning gender: A sociological exploration. Thousand Oaks, CA: Sage, 2011.

[12] Courtenay WH. Constructions of masculinity and their influence on men's well-being: a theory of gender and health. Soc Sci Med 2000;50(10):1385-401.

[13] UN General Assembly. Convention on the elimination of all forms of discrimination against women, 1979. URL: http://www.un.org/womenwatch/daw/cedaw/.

[14] Bruce J, Lloyd CB, Leonard A. Families in focus: New perspectives on mothers, fathers, and children. New York: Population Council, 1995.

[15] Hallman K, Roca E. Reducing the social exclusion of girls. Promoting healthy, safe and productive transitions to adulthood. New York: Population Council, Brief 27, 2007.

[16] Tuwor T, Sossou MA. Gender discrimination and education in West Africa: strategies for maintaining girls in school. Int J Inclusive Educ 2008;12(4):363-79.

[17] United Nations Children's Fund. Harnessing the power of data for girls: Taking stock and looking ahead to 2030. New York: UNICEF, 2016.

[18] Doyal L. Sex, gender, and health: the need for a new approach. BMJ 2001;323(7320):1061.

[19] Fatusi AO, Hindin MJ. Adolescents and youth in developing countries: Health and development issues in context. J Adolescence 2010;33(4):499-508.

[20] Olajubu O. Women in the Yoruba religious sphere. New York: State University of New York Press, 2012.

[21] Jayachandran S. The roots of gender inequality in developing countries. Annu Rev Econ 2015;7(1):63-88.

[22] Mmari KN, Oseni O, Fatusi AO. STI treatment-seeking behaviors among youth in Nigeria: Are there gender differences? Int Perspect Sex Reprod Health 2010;36(2):72-9.

[23] Cohen SA, Richards CL. The Cairo consensus: Population, development and women. Fam Plann Perspect 1994;26(6):272-7.

[24] United Nations Children's Fund. State of the world's children 2012: Children in an Urban World. New York: United Nations Children's Fund, 2012.

[25] Mmari K, Blum R, Sonenstein F, Marshall B, Brahmbhatt H, Venables E, et al. Adolescents' perceptions of health from disadvantaged urban communities: Findings from the WAVE study. Soc Sci Med 2014;104:124-32.

[26] Mmari K, Lantos H, Brahmbhatt H, Delany-Moretlwe S, Lou C, Acharya R, et al. How adolescents perceive their communities: a qualitative study that explores the relationship between health and the physical environment. BMC Public Health 2014;14(1):349. doi:10.1186/1471-2458-14-349.

[27] Olumide AO, Ojengbede OA. The media as a critical determinant of the sexual and reproductive health of adolescents in Ibadan, Nigeria. Sex Reprod Health 2016;8:63-74.

[28] Brislin RW. Research instruments. In: Lonner WJ, Berry JW, eds. Field methods in cross-cultural research. Thousand Oaks, CA: Sage, 1986:137-64.

[29] Olumide AO, Adebayo ES, Ojengbede OA. Using photovoice in adolescent health research: A case-study of the well-being of adolescents in vulnerable environments (WAVE) study in Ibadan, Nigeria. Int J Adolesc Med Health 2016 Oct 14. doi: 10.1515/ijamh-2016-0040.

[30] Computer Software. ATLAS.ti GmbH 7.5.10. Computer software. Berlin: Scientific Sofware Development, 1993-2017.

[31] Glaser B, Strauss A. The discovery of grounded theory: Strategies for qualitative research. Chicago, IL: Aldin, 1967.

[32] Leech NL, Onwuegbuzie AJ. Qualitative data analysis: A compendium of techniques and a framework for selection for school psychology research and beyond. Sch Psychol Q 2008;23(4):587.

[33] Shenton AK. Strategies for ensuring trustworthiness in qualitative research projects. Educ Inform 2004;22(2):63-75.

[34] Abegunde B. Gender inequality: Nigeria and international perspectives. Br J Arts Soc Sci 2014;17(1):165-91.

[35] Mathur S, Greene M, Malhotra A. Too young to wed. The lives, rights, and health of young married girls. Washington, DC: International Center Research Women, 2003.

[36] UNESCO. EFA global monitoring report 2015: Education for All 2000-2015: Achievements and Challenges, 2nd ed. Paris: UNESCO, 2015.

[37] National Population Commission (NPC). Nigeria and ICF International. Nigeria demographic and health survey 2013. Rockville, MD: NPC and ICF International, 2014.

[38] Moore AM, Awusabo-Asare K, Madise N, John-Langba J, Kumi-Kyereme A. Coerced first sex among adolescent girls in sub-Saharan Africa: Prevalence and context. Afr J Reprod Health 2007;11(3):62-82.

[39] World Health Organization. Health for the world's adolescents: A second chance in the second decade: Summary. Geneva: WHO, 2014.

[40] Hallman K, Roca E. Reducing the social exclusion of girls. Promoting healthy, safe and productive transitions to adulthood. New York: Population Council, 2007.

[41] Izugbara CO. Life is not designed to be easy for men: Masculinity and poverty among urban marginalized Kenyan men. Gender Issues 2015;32(2):121-37.

In: Childhood and Adolescence
Editor: Joav Merrick

ISBN: 978-1-53613-574-9

Chapter 7

OVERPARENTING FROM THE PERSPECTIVES OF CHINESE PARENTS AND YOUTHS

Janet TY Leung[1,*], PhD,
Daniel TL Shek[1-5], PhD, FHKPS, BBS, SBS, JP
and Lorrie SL Ng[1], BSocSc

[1]Department of Applied Social Sciences, The Hong Kong Polytechnic University, Hong Kong, PR China,
[2]Centre for Innovative Programmes for Adolescents and Families, The Hong Kong Polytechnic University, Hong Kong, PR China
[3]Department of Social Work, East China Normal University, Shanghai, PR China,
[4]Kiang Wu Nursing College of Macau, Macau, PR China
[5]Division of Adolescent Medicine, Department of Pediatrics, Kentucky Children's Hospital, University of Kentucky College of Medicine, Lexington, Kentucky, US

Overparenting has become an emergent parenting style since the 2000s and blossomed rapidly globally. Unfortunately, empirical studies on

[*] Correspondence: Janet Leung, PhD, Department of Applied Social Sciences, The Hong Kong Polytechnic University, Hunghom, Hong Kong, PR China. Email: janet.leung@polyu.edu.hk.

overparenting are severely lacking particularly in the Chinese context. This study explored the views of Chinese parents and youths on overparenting in Hong Kong. Based on four focus groups involving 23 parents and five young people, eight themes were extracted from the qualitative findings, including close monitoring, intrusion of child's life and direction, strong emphasis on child's academic performance, frequent comparisons on child's achievement with peers, anticipatory problem-solving, overscheduling of child's activities, excessive care, and excessive affective involvement. While some of these themes correspond to overparenting concepts in the Western contexts, some themes are distinctive to the Chinese culture. Theoretical and practical implications of the study are discussed.

INTRODUCTION

Since the 2000s, overparenting has become an emergent parenting style that draws the attention of mass media and the public. Generally speaking, overparenting refers to the phenomenon that parents are over-involved in their children's daily routines and become highly intrusive in their children's lives. It is not surprising to find out that some parents even use Global Positioning System (GPS) to constantly track the whereabouts of their children, asking for special privileges and attention from the teachers for their children, scheduling many interest classes and extracurricular activities for developing the "talents" of their children (1, 2), and actively building up a "greenhouse" for their children to grow up so as to fulfill the dreams of the parents (3).

Conceptually, there are different definitions of overparenting. According to Segrin et al. (4), overparenting refers to "developmentally inappropriate parenting that is driven by parents' overzealous desires to ensure the success and happiness of their children, typically in a way that is construed largely in the parents' terms, and to remove any perceived obstacles to those positive outcomes" (4, p. 238). Similarly, Rousseau and Scharf (5) defined overparenting as "the use of developmentally inappropriate levels of involvement, control, and problem-solving by parents of young adults, and indicates problems in family differentiation, as it emphasizes relatedness while disregarding autonomy" (5, p. 827). Although both definitions emphasize overparenting as a "developmentally inappropriate parenting", they have different foci.

In fact, there is muddiness in defining and conceptualizing overparenting (3). While some researchers posit overparenting as "parenting characteristics taken to an inappropriate degree" (6, p. 405) and focus on the "excessive" levels of parental demandingness, responsiveness, and involvement (7), others look for specific and unique features of overparenting. Regarding the former view (i.e., looking into excessive levels of parenting), Locke et al. (7) conducted a qualitative study to examine the concept of overparenting based on the different aspects of parental demandingness (e.g., demands, supervision, and disciplinary efforts) (8) and responsiveness (e.g., supportive and acquiescence to the child's needs) (8), and suggested that the "excessive" proportion only applied to parental responsiveness but not fully in parental demandingness. While some characteristics of overparenting demonstrate a high level of parental demandingness (e.g., strict parental control, over-scheduling of children's routine), some overparenting behavior does not show high parental demandingness, such as over-protection of children and risk aversion.

Regarding the unique characteristics of overparenting that are different from other parenting styles and practice, Segrin et al. (4, 9) identified four features of overparenting, including anticipatory problem-solving and risk aversion, excessive advice and affective involvement to children, control over children's self-direction, and provision of over-abundant tangible assistance. Garst and Gagnon (10) suggested three main types of overparenting: helicopter parenting, lawnmower parenting, and intrusive parenting. Helicopter parenting refers to parents who excessively shield risks and solve problems for their children; lawnmower parenting means that parents "mow" away from the obstacles from their children's life paths; and intrusive parenting refers to overscheduling and micromanagement of their children's daily routine. An integration of these views suggests some common understanding of overparenting: parents exercise high levels of parental control, care and involvement of their children in their daily routines and life plans, and at the same time they grant less autonomy to them.

As culture plays a crucial role in shaping parenting strategies and adolescent development (11), it is anticipated that there would be differences in the concepts of overparenting between Chinese and Western societies. Particularly, parenting in the Western societies builds on an individualistic perspective that focuses on independence, self-identity, and autonomy of the offspring which is fundamentally different from Chinese parenting that is grounded in a collectivistic perspective focusing on one's responsibilities to bring honor to the family (12, 13).

There are some unique features of Chinese parenting that have relevance to the Chinese concepts of overparenting. First, Chinese parenting is characterized by high levels of demandingness, behavioral control and psychological control over their children (14, 15). Second, good academic performance and personal achievements are stressed by Chinese parents so as to build up family pride (16, 17). Third, parents are highly involved in their children's education and development, and are ready to sacrifice their own needs and interests (18, 19). Fourth, parental control and parental care can coexist from the same parent at the same time (20). These features may serve as an incubator for formulating the Chinese concept of overparenting. Unfortunately, research related to the conceptualization of overparenting is almost non-existent in different Chinese contexts. Computer searches of PsycINFO in April 2017 using the search term "overparenting" produced only 27 publications. The number of citations dropped to "0" when the search term "Chinese" was added. As such, there is a need to explore the conceptions of overparenting in the Chinese context.

Against this background, the study attempted to understand the conception of overparenting from the perspectives of Chinese parents and youths in Hong Kong. Qualitative research using focus group interviews was conducted in the current study. The qualitative research approach explores the interpretive understanding of human experiences and provides more rooms for the exploration and creative synthesis of social reality (21, 22). This allows the participants to voice out the interpretive meanings of overparenting that they have observed and experienced. Among different qualitative data collection strategies, focus group was used to understand the views of parents and adolescents on overparenting. Focus group is "a qualitative research technique used to obtain data about feelings and opinions of a small group of participants about a given problem, experience, service or other phenomenon" (23, p. 414). Krueger (24) suggested that focus group interviews can "tap into human tendencies" (24, p. 10) by capturing the attitudes and perceptions of the participants on a concept or product. This method is particularly sensitive to capture culturally sensitive phenomenon (25). The focus group methodology has been widely used in youth research in Hong Kong (26).

OUR STUDY

In this study, three focus groups of parents and one focus group of youths were recruited. The members of both parent and youth focus groups were recruited from eight children and youth service centers of a non-governmental organization in Hong Kong. There were totally 23 parents participated in the focus groups, forming three focus groups with nine, seven and seven members respectively. Most of them were mothers (n = 22, 95.7%), with one father joining the focus group. The mean age was 45.21 (SD = 5.03). The educational levels of the participants were quite diverse, with five parents (21.7%) havng junior secondary level, five (21.7%) completed Secondary 4 and 5 (Grade 10 and 11), 4 (17.4%) completed Secondary 6 and 7 (Grade 12 and 13), four (17.4%) completed post-secondary education and five (21.7%) completed their undergraduate degree or above. Amongst the respondents, 11 (47.8%) participants were housewives and seven (30.4%) participants were managers or professionals. The majority of the participants were married with their first marriage (n = 18, 78.3%), while three were divorced (13.0%), one was widowed (4.3%) and one had their second marriage (4.3%). The household income also varied among the participants: HK$10,001 - HK$20,000

(US$1,282.2 – US$2,564.1); N = 6 (26.1%); HK$20,001 - HK$30,000 (US$2,564.2 – US$3,846.2); N = 5 (21.7%); HK$60,001 – HK$70,000 (US$7,692.4 – US$8,974.4); N = 4 (17.4%). A higher proportion of parents had two children (N = 12, 52.2%), while 8 (34.8%) parents had only one child. Among their children (N = 41), 29 (70.7%) were boys and 12 (29.3%) were girls. The age of their children ranged from 4 to 25, with the mean age of 14.56 (SD = 4.81).

Regarding the focus group for youths, there were 5 participants. All were females with the mean age at 19.60 (SD = 1.52). Four of them studied in university and one studied in a community college. All lived together with parents. All of them had intact families, with a mean family size of 4.40 (SD = 0.55). Four (80.0%) had one sibling and one had two siblings (20.0%). Three of them (60.0%) had a monthly household income of HK$10,001 - HK$20,000 (US$1,282.2 – US$2,564.1) and the remaining two had the monthly household income (40.0%) of HK$30,001 – HK$40,000 (US$3,846.3 – US$5,128.2).

Data collection was conducted in three children and youth service centers operated by the non-governmental organization. Informed consent from the participants was obtained. The first author was the moderator of the focus group and she led the discussion based on an interview guide (see appendix 1). The participants were encouraged to express their observations, experiences, views and opinions of overparenting in the group. The focus group interviews lasted for approximately one hour. All interviews were audio-recorded under the consent of the participants, and the verbatim was transcribed by student helpers from a university.

A general qualitative orientation was adopted in this study (27). To interpret the qualitative data, thematic analyses using pattern coding was performed. Miles and Huberman (28) suggested that pattern coding is "a way of grouping those summaries into a small number of sets, themes, or constructs ... it's an analog to the cluster-analytic and factor-analytic devices use in statistical analysis" (28, p. 69). To ensure the reliability of the coding, inter-rater reliability check of the selected codes was performed by the first author and the third author.

FINDINGS

In this study, eight themes were extracted from the qualitative data, including close monitoring, the intrusion of child's life and direction, strong emphasis on child's academic performance, frequent comparisons on child's achievement with peers, anticipatory problem-solving, overscheduling of child's activities, excessive care and excessive affective involvement. To assess the inter-rater reliability, the third author coded 96 narratives from parents' and youth's focus groups into eight themes. The first author then recoded the 96 narratives again without knowing the original codes of the third author. The agreement of narratives having the same coding between the first author and the third author was 88 (91.7%). Each theme was discussed in details.

Theme 1: Close monitoring

Both parents and youths identified "close monitoring" as a dimension of overparenting. Overparented parents require the children to strictly follow the rules they had set and report the whereabouts to them constantly. Here are some narratives from the parents and youths:

> "In order to monitor my elder daughter, I used to tell my parents (my child's grandparents) what my daughter needed to do everyday. When my daughter did not meet my requirements or I received any complaints from others, I would give her serious physical punishment. In short, I have set strict rules and regulations for my daughters to follow." (Madam K, parent)
>
> "Wherever they [children] go and whatever they do, they have to ask permissions from their [overparented] parents…Their parents like to regulate what they should or should not do. If the children do something without seeking permission from their parents, or when they make mistakes afterwards, they will be scolded repeatedly all day long." (Madam K, parent)

> "Some adolescents have to go back home within the time limit set by their parents. If they do not do so, they would not be allowed to hang out with friends for one month as a kind of punishment. I have a secondary classmate whose parents are very strict in regulation. If my classmate hanged out with friends at night, her parents would give her non-stop calls and ask the name and telephone number of her friends. They would even call her friends to confirm whether she was really hanging out with them." (Miss E, youth)

Moreover, parents also track their children's whereabouts and behaviors. With the advance of technology, they use the Internet to track the behaviors of their children. Madam M and Madam E had some observations on these parental behaviors:

> "I have heard a mother requesting her daughter to do homework at home and then she went to the gymnasium. Surprisingly, she could check out at the gym room that her daughter was surfing the Facebook at home." (Madam M, parent)
>
> "I witnessed some parents who picked their children up after school even though their children were secondary school students. Moreover, it was not a common practice that parents would accompany their children in school picnic in secondary schools, yet some parents would go to the destination to look for their children." (Madam E, parent)

Theme 2: Intrusion of child's life and direction

Both parents and youths agreed that parents who exercised overparenting intruded into the lives and direction of their children. Parents were particularly sensitive to the social circles of their children. They interfered their children in building relationship with peers. Here are some narratives from the parents:

> "I witnessed a parent restricting her child to make new friends. In a dialogue, a boy told his mom 'Mommy, I want to have lunch with a

classmate.' Then, the mother asked 'How is the academic performance of that classmate? Does he have outstanding academic results? What is his academic ranking in your class?' After the boy told his mother that his classmate was not good in the study, his mother said 'Oh, you should not get along with him then. You should not make friends of low quality. You ought to find other good classmates to have lunch with you.'" (Madam I, parent)

"Just take hanging out with friends at night as an example. A Form 3 student wanted to have their social life and sometimes have dinner with his friends. However, his parents did not allow him to hang out with friends at night in order to protect him from getting along with delinquent friends. If the boy did not follow the rules, his parents might deduct his pocket money. I think this kind of behaviors would affect their children's personal development and the chance to build up interpersonal relationship." (Madam L, parent)

However, the youth informants discussed more deeply on parents' interference of the choices of their study and career. They found that overparented parents would "impose" or "persuade" their desired choice of study and career to their children, regardless of their children's will and interests. Here are some narratives from the youths:

"I remember that I have a schoolmate who chose to study science because of the pressure from her parents. When she was in Form 3, she had to choose the subjects of Humanities or Science for further study. I think she was fond of subjects of Humanities. After communicating with parents, she was requested to study science instead of humanities. Since she had no interest in science at all and encountered lots of unsolved studying difficulties, she could not get the entry ticket to the university finally." (Miss U, youth)

"I have a friend who got fair scores in the public examination and he was qualified to study bachelor of business administration in HKUST [Hong Kong University of Science and Technology] ... His mother wanted him to study Engineering aboard, despite the fact that my friend studied business in secondary school. My friend was very depressed at that time… My friend's mother didn't really care about the true choice of my friend." (Miss D, youth)

To illustrate this point further, the conversation between the moderator and an informant is presented below:

(Y: Miss Y, youth; M: Moderator)

Y: Though I don't want to study in a secondary school for girls only, I had no choice but to do so since my mother already put the school at the first place in the application form. When I had to choose the study stream, I prefer to study Chinese history but my mother wants me to study Accountancy. At last, she successfully persuaded me to study Accountancy. However, I didn't perform well in Accountancy. In my opinion, I am more suitable to study Arts subjects instead of Science and Mathematics subjects.

M: How did your mother persuade you to study a subject that you have no interest in?

Y: Actually, I don't hate Accountancy. But I didn't anticipate that it was a difficult subject and I had to learn complicated calculation. Since my mother said choosing a subject in both Art and Science stream is more beneficial for my future study path, I was convinced to follow her plan.

M: Did parents usually use the reason of practicality or career path to persuade their children when choosing the subjects?

Y: Yes, they did. And they usually ignored the interest and ability of their children.

Theme 3: Strong emphasis on child's academic performance

The emphasis on children's academic performance was salient in Chinese parenting. Indeed, overparented parents paid much effort to boost their children's academic performance. They considered academic performance as the sole indicator to evaluate the future success of their children. There are some narratives from the parents:

"In my community, a lot of parents are very nervous about their children's academic performance. They actively ask their senior students or students of the same grade [from different schools] for past exam papers in order to 'train' their children." (Madam S, parent)

"I think parents who use academic performance as the only indicator to evaluate the success of their children belongs to a group of 'monster parents'. Though some adolescents are not good at study, they have good potentials and outstanding performance in other areas such as sports, art, music etc. However, there are many parents using academic results as the only indicator to evaluate their children. To ensure ideal academic performance, parents would help their children do everything in daily life such as feeding and washing clothes for their children. The only thing the children need to do is to strive for good academic results" (Madam E, parent)

The youth informants expressed their feelings and stresses when parents over-emphasized on their academic performance. Here are some narratives from the youths:

"Nowadays, students attend tutorial classes at a very early stage. I have a primary student [in my tutorial group] who started to have tutorials when he was only a K2 [studying Level 2 in a kindergarten] child... When the boy sometimes got poor academic performance, his parents would show him unhappy face and this made him much more stressful." (Miss E, youth)

"I have a classmate who was very afraid of failing a test or exam since her mother might punish him in a very harsh manner." (Miss Y, youth)

Theme 4: Frequent comparisons of child's achievement with peers

The parent informants observed that parents with overparenting used to compare their children's academic achievement and achievement with their peers. These parents expected that their children would stand out from the peers. They used the peers' results as the reference standard for their children. Here are some narratives:

"I witnessed many parents asking other students about their examination marks and using them to compare with their own children's. I think the examination marks of other children is none of their businesses. The scores sometimes may not reflect the abilities of their children. What they should ask is the difficulty of the examination paper but not the scores of others." (Madam H, parent)

"There are comparisons among parents. Parents used to compare the academic results of their children with others. Though the parents claimed that they only wanted to have an idea about the range of the scores among the classmates, they actually aimed to use the scores for comparison. In my opinion, this value [we need to compare with others] will pass to their children. The children would expect studying hard is for standing out from the rest of class rather than for the attainment of knowledge." (Madam S, parent)

"A story happened in a primary school. Parent A thought his child's masterpiece was better than that of parent B's child. Parent A then came to the school and requested the teacher to add scores to her child's work. She even threatened the teacher if she did not do so, she would report the case to Apple Daily (a local newspaper) or seek help from Law Fan Chiu-fun (former Permanent Secretary for Education and Manpower Bureau). I think almost all school personnel were afraid of parent A." (Madam D, parent)

Theme 5: Anticipatory problem-solving

Parents who exercised overparenting actively "mowed" away any obstacles that might hinder their children's development. Sometimes they were aggressive in solving the anticipated difficulties that their children might encounter, which might offend others and weaken the problem-solving capacities of their children. Here are some narratives from the parent and youth informants:

"In some well-known secondary schools, parents of Form 3 students always ask Form 4 students for studying materials and past exam papers of the core subjects. You can see how active and aggressive the parents are, while their children stand beside and remain passive. I think this kind of parenting practices will nurture adolescents to become weak and passive in problem-solving. Also, it will hinder their personal development in the long run." (Madam S, parent)

"I recognize a parent who liked complaining whenever she felt dissatisfied towards the school practices. For instance, when a teacher made a mistake in a speech in teaching and her child got the meaning wrongly, she would complain to the school principal and even report to the journalists." (Madam M, parent)

"Because of the poor academic performance, my elder brother had to find a job after study. My mother not only helped my brother fill out job application forms, but also accompanied him for job interviews. I think this is an over-parenting practice...Once, I was requested to help my brother line up for a place of study in IVE [Hong Kong Institute of Vocational Education] after the release of his exam results. I think my brother is mature enough to do it by himself ..." (Miss U, youth)

Theme 6: Overscheduling of child's activities

As early as early childhood, parents start to prepare their children by scheduling different learning activities such as language acquisition, talent development, tutoring etc. The parents expect that these learning activities would help their children develop competitiveness in the future. These activities become essential so that the children can "win at the starting line". Here are some narratives from the parent informants:

"One day, I was in a boutique and listened to a parent who has a child studying K1 [Level 1 in a kindergarten], saying that she felt worried about scheduling inadequate activities for her child. She said that some children in the kindergarten would have a schedule of learning different things every hour like dancing, music, abacus calculation etc." (Madam R, parent)

> "I witnessed a girl starting to learn English when she was only three years old. Her parents even hired a teacher to polish her English. The girl had to keep learning many things after school. She is now studying primary school. After school, she has to come back home to learn German and piano. She told me that apart from Friday night, other nights were occupied by different subjects." (Madam G, parent)

However, the children are found exhausted and stressful, and some of them do not feel interested in the activities at all. The youth informants shared their observations:

> "Since many parents nowadays have higher income, they would like their children winning at the starting line. Therefore, they like to arrange many interest and tutorial classes such as phonics and Putonghua for their children. Though my student [in my tutorial group] sometimes get tired of having tutorials, he never speaks to his parents about this feeling. He is a very obedient boy." (Miss E, youth)
>
> "I was a tutor and I observed some parents arranged a lots of activities for their children every week. Even though their children said that they did not want to participate in some interest classes such as dancing and piano, their parents still coerced them to join. I feel like those parents are controlling their children without consideration of their true willingness." (Miss D, youth)

Theme 7: Excessive care

Parents expressed that overparented parents were over-responsive to the needs of the children and adolescents. Rather than training their children to become more independent and responsible for their own self-care, they performed the daily tasks for them, and ensured that their children were taken care of. However, their children were dependent to their parents, and failed to perform the age-appropriate tasks of self-management. Here are some observations from the parent and adolescent informants:

"When my son studied in Primary 6, he once stayed overnight in his friend's house. His friend was excellent in academic performance in a famous school. But my son told me that he did not know how to wash his face and clean his teeth. His father helped him clean his face. He was 12 years old at that time" (Madam E, parent)

"I met a parent who kept taking lunch box to her child for six years in secondary school. The parent even sat beside the adolescent and helped him wipe his sweat off. She kept doing so for six years." (Madam C, parent)

"I met some parents who were rich and thought that their [adult] children earned so little, hence they did not require their children to help out the family expenses. The [adult] daughter got used to ask her mother for pocket money. Recently, she created a Facebook post related to a luxurious meal. She praised her mother and said 'my mother earns money for me to enjoy this luxurious meal. Ha! Ha! Ha!' I think it is too much … The mother even allowed her daughter stay at home without seeking job for several years … I think her parents was nurturing her to become a termite." (Madam L, parent)

"I think my mother gave too much care to my elder brother. She always helped him tidy up the garbage in his room but never asking him to do it by himself. As a result, my brother lacks good self-care ability in his daily life." (Miss U, youth)

Theme 8: excessive affective involvement

Over-parented parents' emotions were easily overwhelmed by the emotions and behaviors of their children. Their over-reaction would exaggerate the consequences of their actions. Here are some narratives from the parent and youth informants:

"Some parents are very nervous and exaggerate minute things. When a child stumbles, just let him stumble. Actually, we get used to stumbling when we were young. There is no need to be so nervous. It is simple, the child learns to be more careful [in the future]. But they would scream, this is very extravagant." (Madam M, parent)

> "My mom is very nervous of my elder brother [emerging adults]. For example, when my elder brother was going to have dinner with his friends, she was very worried and anxious." (Miss U, youth)

DISCUSSION

In order to provide the best for their children and prepare them to win in the "rug rat race" competently, parents make great effort to "train" and "nurture" their children. Overparenting becomes the emergent parenting style that blossom across different ages, races, and regions (3, 29). However, the study of overparenting is at preliminary stage (4, 7). Moreover, culture plays a crucial role in shaping the ecology of parenting and child development (11). Hence, it is essential to understand and study the phenomenon of overparenting with reference to the cultural and contextual characteristics of the community. Against this background, the present study attempted to explore and understand the conceptions of overparenting from the perspectives of Chinese parents and youths in Hong Kong. This is the first known scientific study to understand overparenting in Chinese parents using a qualitative approach. Indeed, this study provides some insights on the understanding and conceptualization of Chinese overparenting, which enhance further studies of overparenting in the Chinese communities.

Based on the Western literature, overparenting is a multi-dimensional construct that parents exercise developmentally inappropriate parenting practices to protect their children from risks by "mowing away" the problems that they anticipate, and intrude into their children's lives and daily routines (4). From the experiences and observations of the parents and youths in this study, overparenting comprises the themes of close monitoring, parental intrusion and anticipatory problem-solving. That is, rather than allowing more space for their children to explore, attempt and learn from trials and errors, overparented parents tend to solve the problems of their children and impose their preferences on their children's lives and directions. Moreover, overparented parents were supposed to be

overprotective towards their children. They show excessive care and excessive affective involvement to their children. Echoed previous research that Chinese parents could be both demanding and responsive to their children (20), parents who exercise overparenting demonstrate close monitoring but at the same time show excessive care in their parenting practice.

Besides, from the qualitative findings based on the Chinese parents and youths, some distinctive features of overparenting were identified, including strong emphasis of academic performance, frequent comparison of child's achievement with peers and over-scheduling of child's activities. These features reflect the emphasis of children's academic performance and personal achievement by the Chinese parents. Exemplary performance in school has been regarded as a familial obligation in compliance with the Chinese socialization value of bringing honor to the family name (30, 31). Chinese parents generally believe that parents play a vital role in the school success of their children by offering parental sacrifice, investment and involvement in the children's learning and schooling (32, 33). Besides, parents used to compare the academic results of their children with their classmates, expecting that their children would excel among the peers. This echoes with the Chinese saying of "*wang zi cheng long*" (i.e., expecting the son to become dragon), with dragon represents "superiority" in the Chinese culture (34). These features would be more prominent in overparenting when parents are more obsessed with children's academic success.

There are theoretical and practical implications of the study. Theoretically, as overparenting is an emergent concept of parenting that is under-researched, especially in the Chinese context, this study revealed the concept and dimensions of Chinese overparenting from the perspectives of parents and youths in Hong Kong. The findings provide important insights for family researchers and scholars in the conceptions and themes of this emergent parenting style, which may be different from the Western conceptions of overparenting. This helps us develop an indigenous model of Chinese overparenting in the social science literature.

Methodologically, the conceptualization of Chinese overparenting may help researchers develop an indigenous measurement in assessing overparenting applicable to the Chinese communities. Yang (35) suggested that in constructing a new measurement of overparenting, there is a need to do a qualitative pilot study to capture the native meanings and features of phenomenon. As such, this study taped the indigenous views of overparenting from parents and youths, which facilitated the construction and development of a measurement of Chinese overparenting. The availability of a validated indigenous measurement would further enhance future research on examining the relationships among overparenting, family dynamics and adolescent development in the Chinese contexts.

Practically, the themes extracted from the qualitative findings provide important cues for family practitioners and helping professionals to identify families that exercise overparenting and provide timely responses and service for the families. In fact, there are studies in the United States showing that overparenting negatively influenced psychological wellbeing (6) and positively predicted depression and anxiety (5, 9, 36) of emerging adults. Besides, there is empirical evidence that overparenting had adverse effects on parent-child communication, which in turn decreased the family satisfaction of adolescents (4). Hence, it is important for the family practitioners and helping professionals to enhance the awareness of the parents through parental education programs.

Although this is a pioneer study on the structure of over-parenting in a Chinese context, there are several limitations of the study. First, the study was based on the qualitative data collected from focus groups of general parents and youth in Hong Kong. It would be more insightful if parents and youths who are involved in overparenting were recruited. They would provide more information on their actual experiences on overparenting. Second, only one group of youths (all were females) was recruited in the study. Besides, there is a need to explore the views and experiences from the male youths. Similarly, as most parent informants were mothers, the perspective from fathers on overparenting was ignored but indeed important and insightful to understand the concepts of overparenting because parent gender differences were commonly found in the scientific literature (37, 38). Third, parents and youths were recruited in Hong Kong. There may be contextual differences between Hong Kong and other

Chinese communities (e.g., mainland China and Chinese communities in the United States). Hence, further studies should be conducted in other Chinese communities. Last but not the least, more qualitative data collection techniques such as case interviews can help to understand the subjective experiences of the informants more deeply.

ACKNOWLEDGMENTS

This research was financially supported by the Departmental General Research Fund of The Hong Kong Polytechnic University (G-UA9S). This chapter is a re-published work based on an article published in the International Journal of Child and Adolescent Health 2018; 11(3) issue.

APPENDIX 1. INTERVIEW GUIDE OF THE FOCUS GROUP

1. What does "overparenting" mean to you? What are the features that you perceive in "overparenting"?
2. Have you experienced (exercised) overparenting in your family? What are the practices? Can you illustrate the practices with examples?
3. Have your ever observed parents who exercised overparenting? What were the practices? Can you illustrate the practices with examples?
4. Who used to exercise overparenting, father or mother or both? Are there any differences between paternal overparenting and maternal overparenting? What are the differences?
5. What were the responses of the children on overparenting?
6. What are the possible outcomes of the children when parents exercise overparenting?
7. What are the factors that contribute to overparenting?

8. What are the general demographic characteristics of the families that exercise overparenting? Does overparenting happen mostly in families having high socio-economic status, and/or in families with lone child?

REFERENCES

[1] Lareau A. Unequal childhoods. Berkeley, CA: University California Press, 2003.
[2] Yip MY. Helicopter parents. Hong Kong: World Press, 2011. [Chinese]
[3] Leung JTY, Busiol D. Adolescents growing up in a "Greenhouse": A literature review. Int J Child Adolesc Health 2016;9(4):413-22.
[4] Segrin C, Woszidlo A, Givertz M, Bauer A, Taylor Murphy M. The association between overparenting, parent-child communication, and entitlement and adaptive traits in adult children. Fam Relat 2012;61(2):237-52.
[5] Rousseau S, Scharf M. "I will guide you" The indirect link between overparenting and young adults' adjustment. Psychiatry Res 2015;228:826-34.
[6] LeMoyne T, Buchanan T. Does "hovering" matter? Helicopter parenting and its effect on well-being. Sociol Spectr 2011;31(4):399-418.
[7] Locke JY, Campbell MA, Kavanagh D. Can a parent do too much for their child? An examination by parenting professionals of the concept of overparenting. Aust J Guid Couns 2012;22(2):249-65.
[8] Baumrind D. Parenting styles and adolescent development. In: Brooks-Gunn J, Lerner R, Peterson AC, eds. The encyclopedia of adolescence. New York: Garland, 1991:746-58.
[9] Segrin C, Woszidlo A, Givertz M, Montgomery N. Parent and child traits associated with overparenting. J Soc Clin Psychol 2013;32(6):569-95.
[10] Garst BA, Gagnon RJ. Exploring overparenting within the context of youth development programs. J Youth Dev 2015;10(1):6-18.
[11] Bornstein MH, Cheah CSL. The place of "culture and parenting" in the ecological contextual perspective on developmental science. In: Rubin KH, Chung OB, eds. Parenting beliefs, behaviors, and parent-child relationship. New York: Taylor Francis, 2006:3-34.
[12] Leung JTY. Cultural family beliefs, maternal sacrifice, and adolescent psychological competence in Chinese poor single-mother families. Soc Dev 2017. doi:10.1111/sode.12239.
[13] Shek DTL. Chinese family research: Puzzles, progress, paradigms, and policy implications. J Fam Issues 2006;27(3):275-84.

[14] Chao RK. Beyond parental control and authoritarian parenting style: Understanding Chinese parenting through the cultural notion of training. Child Dev 1994;65(4):1111-9.

[15] Shek DTL. A longitudinal study of perceived parental psychological control and psychological well-being in Chinese adolescents in Hong Kong. J Clin Psychol 2007;63(1):1-22.

[16] Blair SL, Qian Z. Family and Asian students' educational performance: A consideration of diversity. J Fam Issues 1998;19(4):355-74.

[17] Chao RK, Sue S. Chinese parental influence and their children's school success: a paradox in the literature on parenting styles. In: Lau S. ed. Growing up the Chinese way: Chinese child and adolescent development. Hong Kong: Chinese University Press, 1996;93-120.

[18] Leung JTY, Shek DTL. Are family processes related to achievement motivation of Chinese adolescents experiencing economic disadvantage in Hong Kong? Int J Disabil Hum Dev 2013;12(2):115-25.

[19] Leung JTY, Shek DTL. Parenting for resilience: Family processes and psychosocial competence of Chinese adolescents experiencing economic disadvantage in Hong Kong. Int J Disabil Hum Dev 2013;12(2):127-37.

[20] Lau S, Cheung PC. Relationships between Chinese adolescents' perception of parental control and organization and their perception of parental warmth. Dev Psychol 1987;23(5):726-9.

[21] Leung JTY, Shek DTL. Qualitative and quantitative approaches in the study of poverty and adolescent development: Separation or integration? Int J Adolesc Med Health 2011;23(2):115-21.

[22] Patton MQ. Qualitative evaluation and research methods. Thousand Oaks, CA: Sage, 1990.

[23] Basch CE. Focus group interview: An underutilized research technique for improving theory and practice in health education. Health Educ Q 1987;14:411-48.

[24] Krueger RA. Focus groups: A practical guide for applied research, 2nd ed. Newbury Park, CA: Sage, 1994.

[25] Kitzinger J. Introducing focus groups. BMJ 1995;311(7000):299-302.

[26] Shek DTL. The use of focus groups in programme evaluation: Experience based on the Project P.A.T.H.S. in a Chinese context. In: Barber R, Morgan D, eds. A new era of focus group research. Hampshire: Palgrave MacMillan, in press.

[27] Shek DTL, Tang VMY, Han XY. Evaluation of evaluation studies using qualitative research methods in the social work literature (1990-2003): Evidence that constitutes a wake-up call. Res Soc Work Pract 2005;15(3):180-94.

[28] Miles MB, Huberman AM. Qualitative data analysis. Thousand Oaks. CA: Sage, 1994.

[29] Gibbs N. The growing backlash against overparenting. Time Magazine [internet] URL: http://www.time.com/time/magazine/article/0,9171,1940697,00.html.

[30] Chao RK. The parenting of immigrant Chinese and European American mothers: Relations between parenting styles, socialization goals, and parental practices. J Appl Dev Psychol 2000;21(2):233-48.
[31] Kim U, Chun M. Educational "success" of Asian Americans: An indigenous perspective. J Appl Dev Psychol 1994;15(3):329-43.
[32] Chao RK. Chinese and European American mothers' beliefs about the role of parenting in children's school success. J Cross Cult Psychol 1996;27(4):403-23.
[33] Leung JTY, Shek DTL. "All I can do for my child" --- Development of the Chinese Parental Sacrifice for Child's Education Scale. Int J Disabil Hum Dev 2011;10(3):201-8.
[34] Leung JTY, Shek DTL. Expecting my child to become "Dragon": Development of the Chinese Parental Expectation on Child's Future Scale. Int J Disabil Hum Dev 2011:10(3):257-65.
[35] Yang KS. Towards an indigenous Chinese psychology: A selective review of methodological, theoretical, and empirical accomplishments. Chinese J Psychol 1999;41(2):181-211.
[36] Schiffrin HH, Liss M, Miles-McLean H, Geary KA, Erchull MJ, Tashner T. Helping or hovering? The effects of helicopter parenting on college students' well-being. J Child Fam Stud 2014;23(3):548-57.
[37] Leung JTY, Shek DTL. Parental differences in family processes in Chinese families experiencing economic disadvantage. Géneros 2012;1(3):271-99.
[38] Shek DTL. Perceived parental control and parent-child relational qualities in early adolescents in Hong Kong: Parent gender, child gender and grade differences. Sex Roles 2008;58:666-81.

In: Childhood and Adolescence
Editor: Joav Merrick
ISBN: 978-1-53613-574-9

Chapter 8

MOTHERS' ATTRIBUTIONS IN THE RELATIONSHIP BETWEEN YOUNG CHILDREN'S TEMPERAMENT AND PARENTING STRESS

Melissa Middleton, PhD and Kimberly Renk*, PhD
Tulane University School of Medicine, New Orleans, Louisiana, US
Department of Psychology, University of Central Florida,
Orlando, Florida, US

Although extensive research has been devoted to understanding mother-child relationships, few studies have examined mothers' differential attributions as mediators in the relationship between young children's temperament and mothers' parenting stress. As a result, the current study examined the relationships among young children's temperament, mothers' attributions, mothers' parenting stress, and young children's behavior problems using the responses of mothers who were raising children between the ages of 3 and 6 years. Using correlation and

* Correspondence: Kimberly Renk, PhD, Department of Psychology, University of Central Florida, POBox 161390, Orlando, FL 32816, United States.
Email: Kimberly.Renk@ucf.edu.

regression analyses, results of this study suggested that these variables were interrelated significantly. Regression results also indicated that mothers' attributions mediated the relationship between young children's temperament and mothers' parenting stress. Further, mothers' attributions appeared to be important predictors of their young children's behavior problems. Such findings suggested that interventions would benefit from targeting mothers' attributions of their young children and mothers' reflective functioning as well as the relationships among mothers' attributions, parenting stress, and young children's behavior problems.

INTRODUCTION

Although extensive research has examined the contributions made by mothers and their young children to the mother-young child relationship and to young children's emotional and behavioral outcomes (1), less research has examined mothers' attributions about their young children, even though such attributions may be informative in the context of parenting interventions. In particular, mothers' attributions have been related closely to how mothers perceive and respond to their young children's behavior (2). Further, mothers' attributions may be related uniquely to mothers' own characteristics (like parenting stress) (3) and to those of their young children (e.g., temperament) (1, 4). Given their potential importance, this study examined mothers' attributions as mediators in the relationship between young children's temperament and mothers' parenting stress and as predictors of young children's behavior problems.

Young children's temperament

Young children's temperament is an important starting point in understanding what transpires in the mother-young child relationship. Many researchers consider temperament to be young children's biologically based, early appearing emotional and behavioral dispositions (1). Further, temperament includes young children's propensities toward emotional reactivity and self-regulation (5), with such propensities being considered innate (6) and stable (7). Initially, temperament was described using three broad categories that included easy, difficult, and slow-to-warm children (8). These categories still are used to simply characterize temperament. For example, young children who have difficult temperaments are active, rigid, unaffectionate, and aversive, whereas young children who have easy temperaments are flexible, positive, and affectionate (9). Nonetheless, temperament is much more complex than is portrayed with this conceptualization (e.g., there are nine temperament characteristics) (10).

Overall, however, young children's temperament is related to the ways in which they react to others and others react to them (6, 11, 12). For example, Bowlby (11) stated that infants with easy temperaments are more likely to have mothers who develop positive, effective parenting behaviors; however, infants with difficult temperaments are more likely to have mothers who develop negative, unfavorable parenting behaviors. In addition, mothers of infants with difficult temperaments are at risk for depression (13), which may exacerbate negative parenting behaviors and parenting stress. Further, young children's temperaments are related to mothers' perceptions of their young children (12). For example, mothers' negative attributions for children's behavior increase when they observe difficult temperament characteristics (14). Thus, young children's temperament may be related to mothers' attributions, which may be related to mothers' parenting behaviors.

Although these relationships appear commonsensical, little research has examined collectively young children's temperament, mothers' attributions, mothers' parenting stress, and young children's behavior problems. Certainly, research noted that parents' reactions to their children's temperaments have important implications for children's emotional and behavioral development (15). Research has yet to explain this relationship, however.

Parents' attributions of young children's behavior

Much of the research regarding attributions addressed generally how individuals perceive and evaluate their environment in order to explain events and behaviors (16). Given this explanation, attributions also can be considered a vital part of familial interactions and relationships (16). In fact, Miller (16) stated that there are three overlapping categories of parents' attributions. The first category consists of the immediate reasons for children's behavior (i.e., personality traits, effort, and ability), the second category refers to long-term explanations for children's behavior (i.e., the role of parents' versus children's genes in shaping children's development), and the third category consists of locus of control, stability, and controllability over the parent-child interaction (17). Given that parents' cognitions were deemed important to understanding parent-child interactions (18), this study examined the attributions of children's personality traits, locus of control, and controllability over parent-child interactions. These attributions all can be understood from mothers' points of view, making mothers' reports important for this study.

With regard to these different attributions, parents' attributions regarding children's personality traits (i.e., trait conceptions) refer to the way in which parents perceive their children's personality and are related to parents' expectations for their children's future behavior (19). Research suggested that behavioral observations lead to trait inferences that are stored in memory. These inferences are related to future processing of children's behavior and may lead to biased perceptions (20). For example, research indicated that parents' negative representations of their children's traits are related to their interpretations of and responses to their children's behaviors (19).

Further, locus of control refers to mothers' beliefs that they can influence their children's behavior (internal locus of control) or not (external locus of control) (21). In fact, parents' beliefs regarding their own general abilities are related to their views of parenting and their children's behaviors (16, 22). For example, parents with an external locus of control display less effective parenting behaviors and more authoritarian parenting

(22). In contrast, parents who have an internal locus of control are more likely to use authoritative parenting when confronted with children's uncontrollable, negative behavior (23) and to provide nonverbal warmth toward their children (24).

In contrast, attributions encompassing controllability over parent-child interactions refer to the power or control capability that is attributed to parents versus children. In particular, parents who feel that they have low control over their children's behavior are more likely to be distressed by their children's negative behavior (25), to display harsh, negative parenting, and to subsequently promote and maintain coercive parent-child interactions (26). Conversely, Rubin and Mills (27) suggested that, when parents consider children's behavior to be out of their children's control, parents are less likely to respond negatively, as parents believe that these behaviors cannot be corrected, even if they respond. As these attributions are related to mothers' responses to their children, they also may be related to mothers' parenting stress (18).

Parenting stress

Parenting stress describes the stress that occurs from the demands of being a parent (29). In fact, Abidin (30) suggested that parenting stress results from children's characteristics (e.g., temperament), parents' characteristics (e.g., depression), and demographic life stress. For example, research indicated that children's temperament may either buffer against or increase parenting stress, with difficult child temperament exacerbating parenting stress (8). Further, research linked parenting stress to negative parenting practices and parent-child interactions (31). Fischer (32) also suggested that it may be parents' attention to negative aspects of their children's behavior (33), increased negative attributions about children's behavior (26), and parents being more susceptible to children's negative behavior (34) that explain the relationship between parenting stress and negative parenting behaviors. Thus, mothers' attributions may be related closely to mothers' parenting stress and to young children's behavior problems. A better understanding of these relationships may inform interventions that alleviate parenting stress and young children's behavior problems.

Young children's internalizing and externalizing behavior problems

Nonetheless, few studies examined young children's temperament, mothers' attributions, mothers' parenting stress, and young children's behavior problems collectively. Such collective relationships, with a particular focus on mothers' attributions, may be important to understanding young children's behavior problems. When conceptualizing young children's behavior problems, a dichotomy of problems often is considered. In particular, internalizing behavior problems are characterized by withdrawal, depression, inhibition, and anxiety (35), whereas externalizing behavior problems are characterized by marked noncompliance, frequent aggression, temper tantrums, impulsivity, hyperactivity, and poor frustration tolerance (36). Both internalizing and externalizing behavior problems are relatively stable from early childhood into later development (37), suggesting that understanding their precursors is important.

Certainly, research demonstrated that children's own contributions are important to the development of internalizing and externalizing behavior problems beginning as early as infancy (8). In fact, many studies documented relationships between children's early temperament and their display of later behavior problems (38, 39). For example, children who have difficult temperaments are less successful at self-regulating emotions and are more likely to display behavior problems (4). Research indicated, however, that only a subset of children who have difficult temperaments display long-term internalizing and externalizing behavior problems (37). Thus, it is important to consider mothers' attributions of their young children and mothers' parenting stress, in the context of young children's temperament, as additional predictors of young children's behavior problems. For example, young children's temperament may be related to mothers' attributions and the way in which they think about and behave toward their young children (27, 40). Subsequently, these attributions may be related to young children's behavior problems.

The current study

Given the potential collective relationships among young children's temperament, mothers' attributions, mothers' parenting stress, and young children's behavior problems, it is important to focus on explaining how these variables are related and how they can be used to better parenting interventions. It was expected that mothers' attributions would be associated with young children's temperament, mothers' parenting stress, and young children's behavior problems. Further, it was anticipated that mothers' attributions would mediate the relationship between young children's temperament and mothers' parenting stress. Finally, it was expected that young children's temperament, mothers' attributions, and mothers' parenting stress would make unique contributions to predicting young children's behavior problems. In this study, each temperament dimension that was examined was rated on a continuum ranging from a difficult characterization (e.g., higher activity level) to an easy characterization (e.g., lower activity level).

OUR STUDY

Participants in this study were 81 mothers of children who were attending preschools in Central Florida. The suggested sample size for a multiple regression analysis ($p < .05$) with six independent variables (i.e., the most complex analysis in this study) and a statistical power of .80 is 97 participants in order to detect a medium effect size ($R = .30$) and 45 participants in order to detect a large effect size ($R = .50$) (41). As a result, the sample size for this study should be sufficient. Although data were collected from 27 fathers, only analyses for mothers are reported in this study due to the relatively low number of participating fathers.

In this sample, mothers ranged in age from 18 to 48 years (M = 31.86 years, SD = 6.80 years). The majority of mothers were Caucasian (70.4%). The remainder reported that they were African American (9.9%), Hispanic American (9.9%), Asian American (2.5%), or from some "Other" ethnic background (7.4%). The majority of these mothers were married (59.3%), with the remaining mothers varying in their marital status (i.e., 23.5% were single, 8.6% were divorced, 6.2% were remarried, and 2.5% were widowed). Their level of education (i.e., 3.7% had a high school diploma or less, 1.2% had vocational training, 38.3% had some college, 33.3% had a Bachelor's degree, 18.5% had a Master's degree, and 4.9% had a Doctoral degree) and yearly household income (i.e., 64.2% made less than $30,000, 24.6% made between $30,000 and $60,000, 7.4% made between $60,000 and $90,000, and 2.5% made over $90,000) varied. These mothers provided ratings regarding their young children (50.0% of whom were male, and 50.0% of whom were female), who ranged in age from 3 to 6 years (M = 4.17 years, SD = 1.04 years).

Measures

Young Children's Temperament. The Dimensions of Temperament Scale-Revised for Children (DOTS-R) (10) was used as a measure of mothers' ratings of their young children's temperament. The DOTS-R is a 54-item questionnaire that assesses nine temperament characteristics using a 4-point scale that ranges from 'Usually True' to 'Usually False.' High scores on each scale reflect higher levels of each temperament characteristic. Based on previous literature (9), the temperament characteristics of Activity Level-General, Flexibility/Rigidity, and Mood Quality were used in this study, as they distinguish between difficult and easy temperament. In a previous study (10), the internal consistency of these scales (Activity Level = .84, Flexibility/Rigidity = .79, and Mood Quality = .91) was adequate. Similarly, the internal consistency of Activity

Level (.91), Flexibility/Rigidity (.82), and Mood Quality (.82) was adequate in the current study.

Attributions. The Child Trait Rating Scale (CTRS) (42) was used as a measure of mothers' child trait conceptions. The CTRS consists of 15 traits that were collected from several self-concept measures and that assess parents' global trait perceptions of their children. Each trait is rated on a 7-point Likert scale, with positive and negative poles of each trait at the endpoints. Higher total CTRS scores reflect positive trait conceptions. A previous study reported a Cronbach alpha of .76 (42). In the current study, the internal consistency also was adequate (.78).

The Parenting Locus of Control Scale–Short Form (PLOC-SF) (43) was used as a measure of mothers' locus of control. The PLOC-SF is a 25-item questionnaire that measures the degree to which parents believe that they can influence their children's behavior. It is a shortened form of the Parenting Locus of Control Scale (PLOC) (44). Each item is rated using a 5-point scale that ranges from 'Strongly Agree' to 'Strongly Disagree.' Higher total scores indicate higher internal locus of control. Rayfield, Eyberg, Boggs, and Roberts (45) reported a Cronbach alpha of .79 for the total score. In this study, the internal consistency for this total score also was adequate (.80).

The Parent Attribution Test (PAT) (46) was used as a measure of mothers' attributions of controllability over parent-child interactions. Each of the items on the PAT is rated using a 7-point scale that ranges from 'Not At All Important' to 'Very Important.' The PAT provides measures of the control attributed to adults for caregiving success (ACS) and failure (ACF) and to children for caregiving success (CCS) and failure (CCF). The composite of the ACF and CCF scores constitutes a measure of perceived control over failure (PCF). The composite of the ACS and CCS scores creates a measure of perceived control over success (PCS). In this study, the PCF score, which had adequate internal consistency (.74), was used.

Parenting Stress. The Parenting Stress Index-Short Form (PSI-SF) (30) was used as a measure of mothers' parenting stress. The PSI-SF is a 36-item self-report measure that is derived from the original Parenting Stress

Index (PSI) (29). Each item on the PSI-SF is rated on a 5-point scale that ranges from 'Strongly Agree' to 'Strongly Disagree.' This measure has three subscales (i.e., a Parent Domain that assesses parents' stress in the parent role, a Child Domain that assesses parents' expectations of their children, and a Difficult Child Domain that assesses children's behavioral characteristics). These subscales can be combined into a total parenting stress score, with higher scores indicating higher levels of stress. In a previous study, the PSI-SF had acceptable psychometric properties (30). In the current study, the internal consistency of the total parenting stress score was good (.91).

Young Children's Behavior Problems. The Child Behavior Checklist (CBCL) (47, 48) was used as a measure of mothers' ratings of their young children's behavior problems. Mothers completed either the 1.5- to 5-year old version or the 6- to 18-year old version, depending on the age of their young child. In both versions, mothers rate items on a 3-point scale that ranges from 'Not True' to 'Very True or Often True.' These ratings then were used to derive T scores for young children's behavior problems, allowing comparability across the different versions of the scale. In the current study, the Internalizing Problems and Externalizing Problems scales were used. The CBCL has sound psychometric properties and is noted to differentiate between children who are clinically referred and those who are not. The CBCL is one of the most widely used measures of children's emotional and behavioral functioning (47, 48).

Demographics. Finally, mothers completed a brief demographics questionnaire that asked them to provide information about themselves and their children (e.g., age, occupation).

Procedure

After receiving approval from the Institutional Review Board, the directors of 40 preschools in Central Florida were contacted via telephone and/or e-mail to explain the study and request permission for their schools' participation. Following receipt of permission from 28 preschool directors, young children at each preschool were given a recruitment letter for the study and a consent form for their parents to complete. Parents returned consent forms directly to their young children's teachers, and investigators collected the forms from the preschool directors. Investigators then provided research packets and a debriefing form to those parents who agreed to participate. Parents completed the research packets at home and returned them in sealed envelopes provided by the investigators to their young children's preschool director. Investigators then collected the completed research packets for inclusion in this study.

In addition, researchers recruited participants through an announcement printed in an on-line university newsletter that is distributed via e-mail to university staff and students. This announcement was included in the newsletter one day per week for approximately eight weeks. The announcement instructed potential participants to contact the investigators in order to obtain a full description of the study. After contacting the investigators, each potential participant was mailed a recruitment letter for the study, a consent form, a research packet, and a debriefing form. Parents completed the packet at home and returned it via a postage paid envelope to the investigators. Overall, 37 participants were recruited through participating Central Florida preschools, and 44 participants were recruited through the university newsletter. The participants of this study were not compensated for their participation. All data were analyzed using pairwise deletion to minimize the loss of data included in analyses.

OUR FINDINGS

To put mothers' ratings on each of the measures into context, means and standard deviations were calculated and are presented in Table 1. With regard to temperament, mothers reported that, on average, their young children were moderately active, had a somewhat flexible behavioral style, and had a more positive quality of mood. With regard to attributions, mothers reported having more positive child trait conceptions and a more internal locus of control. Mothers also rated parents and children as having relatively similar levels of control over unsuccessful parent-child interactions. Further, mothers reported that, on average, they were experiencing moderate levels of parenting stress. Finally, mothers rated their children as experiencing nonclinical levels of internalizing and externalizing behavior problems, on average.

Table 1. Descriptive statistics for mother's ratings of the variables of interest

Variables (Range)	*M*	*SD*
Temperament		
Child Activity Level (7-28)	17.77	5.02
Child Flexibility (5-20)	15.36	3.20
Child Mood (7-28)	26.33	2.98
Attributions		
Child Trait Conception (15-105)	82.16	11.62
Parental Locus of Control (25-125)	95.07	12.07
Adult Controllability (5-35)	25.77	3.73
Child Controllability (5-35)	22.25	3.40
Parenting Stress		
Stress (36-180)	67.60	16.87
Child Behavior Problems		
Internalizing Behavior Problems	44.73	9.47
Externalizing Behavior Problems	44.76	9.77

Correlational analyses

Correlations were calculated to examine the relationships among young children's temperament, mothers' attributions, mothers' parenting stress, and young children's behavior problems. See Table 2 for the results of these correlational analyses. Results suggested that mothers who rated their young children as having less flexible behavioral styles also reported that their children had higher activity levels and less positive mood quality. With regard to young children's temperament and mothers' attributions, mothers who rated their young children as having greater activity level also reported having less positive child trait conceptions and a more external locus of control. In addition, mothers who rated their young children as having a more flexible behavioral style reported more positive child trait attributions and a more internal locus of control. Lastly, mothers who rated their young children as having a more positive mood quality also endorsed a more internal locus of control. With regard to young children's temperament and parenting stress, mothers who rated their young children as displaying a greater general activity level, a less flexible behavioral style, and a less positive quality of mood reported higher parenting stress. Mothers who endorsed less positive child trait conceptions and a more external locus of control also reported higher parenting stress.

Finally, with regard to young children's internalizing behavior problems, mothers who rated their young children as having a less flexible behavioral style and a less positive mood quality reported that their young children had higher levels of internalizing behavior problems. Further, mothers who endorsed less positive child trait conceptions and an external locus of control rated their young children as having higher levels of internalizing behavior problems. With regard to young children's externalizing behavior problems, mothers who rated their young children as displaying a higher activity level, a less flexible behavioral style, and a less positive mood quality reported that their young children had higher levels of externalizing behavior problems. Further, mothers who endorsed less positive child trait conceptions and an external locus of control rated their young children as having higher levels of externalizing behavior problems. Mothers who endorsed higher parenting stress also rated their young children as experiencing higher levels of internalizing and externalizing behavior problems.

Table 2. Correlations among Mothers' ratings of temperament, attributions, parenting stress and behavior problems

Variables	1	2	3	4	5	6	7	8	9	10
1. Child Activity Level	-									
2. Child Flexibility	-.38**	-								
3. Child Mood	-.16	.53***	-							
4. Parent Locus of Control	-.30**	.49***	.28*	-						
5. Child Trait Rating Rating	-.25*	.29**	.12	.43***	-					
6. Adult Controllability over parent-child interactions	-.11	.03	-.12	.20	.09	-				
7. Child Controllability over parent-child interactions	.06	-.03	-.07	-.02	.15	.19	-			
8. Parenting Stress	.31**	-.42***	-.28*	-.68***	-.60***	-.10	-.03	-		
9. Child Internalizing	.18	-.49***	-.28*	-.31**	-.43***	.11	.07	.39**	-	
10. Child Externalizing	.38**	-.32**	-.26*	-.46***	-.44***	-.05	-.12	.45***	.52***	-

Note. * $p < .05$; ** $p < .01$; *** $p < .001$.

Mothers' attributions as mediators of temperament and parenting stress

To examine mothers' attributions as mediators in the relationship between young children's temperament and mothers' parenting stress, regression analyses were conducted using each of the attributions that were related significantly to young children's temperament and mothers' parenting stress (i.e., child trait conceptions and locus of control, as controllability over parent-child interactions was not related significantly). Based on Baron and Kenny (49), establishing a mediation model requires several findings. In a series of regression equations, young children's temperament must predict mothers' attributions and mothers' parenting stress. Finally, the relationship between young children's temperament and mothers' parenting stress must decrease to non-significance in the presence of mothers' attributions, indicating that mothers' attributions are acting as mediators. Results of these analyses are presented in Table 3.

Mothers' child trait attributions

When examining child trait conceptions as a mediator in the relationship between young children's flexibility and parenting stress, mothers' ratings of young children's flexibility predicted significantly mothers' child trait conceptions. Next, young children's flexibility predicted significantly mothers' parenting stress. Then, collectively, mothers' ratings of young children's flexibility and child trait conceptions predicted significantly mothers' parenting stress. In particular, when entered first, young children's flexibility predicted significantly parenting stress. When mothers' child trait conceptions were added to this equation, however, young children's flexibility decreased in significance when predicting parenting stress. Thus, mothers' child trait conceptions partially mediated the relationship between young children's flexibility and parenting stress. The mediational value of mothers' child trait conceptions was confirmed with a significant Sobel Test ($z = 3.48$, $p < .001$).

Table 3. Mediational regression analyses for mothers' ratings

Regression/Variables	Beta	*t*	*p*
Mediator: Child Trait Ratings			
Child Flexibility Predicting Child Trait Ratings: F (1, 79) = 7.44, $p < .01$ $r^2 = .09$			
Child Flexibility	.29	2.73	.01
Child Flexibility and Child Trait Ratings Predicting Parenting Stress: F (2, 78) = 30.54, $p < .001$, $r^2 = .43$			
Child Flexibility	-.29	-3.23	.002
Child Trait Ratings	-.52	-5.85	.001
Child Activity Level Predicting Child Trait Ratings: F (1, 79) = 5.38, $p < .05$, $r^2 = .05$			
Child Activity Level	-.25	-2.32	.05
Child Activity Level and Child Trait Ratings Predicting Parenting Stress: F (2, 78) = 25.14, $p < .001$, $r^2 = .38$			
Child Activity Level	.17	1.89	.06
Child Trait Ratings	-.56	-6.13	.001
Child Mood Quality Predicting Child Trait Ratings: F (1, 79) = 1.05, $p < .31$, $r^2 = .01$			
Child Mood Quality	.12	1.03	.31
Mediator: Parental Locus of Control			
Child Flexibility Predicting Parenting Locus of Control: F (1, 79) = 24.38, $p < .001$, $r^2 = .23$			
Child Flexibility	.49	4.94	.001
Child Flexibility and Parental Locus of Control Predicting Parenting Stress: F (2, 80) = 35.81, $p < .001$, $r^2 = .47$			
Child Flexibility	-.14	-1.52	.13
Parental Locus of Control	-.61	-6.54	.001
Child Activity Level Predicting Parenting Locus of Control: F (1, 79) = 6.98, $p < .001$ $r^2 = .47$			
Child Activity Level	-.29	-2.64	.01
Child Activity Level and Parental Locus of Control Predicting Parenting Stress: F (2, 80) = 35.84, $p < .001$, $r^2 = .23$			
Child Activity Level	.13	1.53	.13
Parental Locus of Control	-.64	-7.55	.001
Child Mood Quality Predicting Parental Locus of Control: F (1, 79) = 6.80, $p < .05$, $r^2 = .07$			
Child Mood Quality	.28	2.61	.01
Child Mood Quality and Parental Locus of Control Predicting Parenting Stress: F (2, 78) = 34.84, $p < .001$, $r^2 = .46$			
Child Mood Quality	-.10	-1.13	.26
Parental Locus of Control	-.65	-7.62	.001

When examining child trait conceptions as a mediator in the relationship between young children's activity level and parenting stress, mothers' ratings of young children's activity level predicted significantly mothers' child trait conceptions. Next, young children's activity level predicted significantly mothers' parenting stress. Then, collectively, mothers' ratings of young children's activity level and child trait conceptions predicted significantly mothers' parenting stress. In particular, when entered first, young children's activity level predicted significantly parenting stress. When mothers' child trait conceptions were added to this equation, however, only mothers' child trait conceptions were a significant predictor of parenting stress. Thus, mothers' child trait conceptions fully mediated the relationship between young children's activity level and parenting stress. The mediational value of mothers' child trait conceptions was confirmed with a significant Sobel Test ($z = -2.64$, $p < .01$).

Lastly, when examining child trait conceptions as a mediator in the relationship between young children's quality of mood and parenting stress, mothers' ratings of young children's mood quality did not predict significantly their child trait conceptions. As this relationship was not significant, mediation was not possible, and further analyses were not completed.

Mothers' locus of control attributions

When examining mothers' ratings of locus of control as a mediator in the relationship between young children's flexibility and parenting stress, mothers' ratings of young children's flexibility predicted significantly mothers' locus of control. Next, mothers' ratings of young children's flexibility predicted significantly mothers' parenting stress. Then, collectively, mothers' ratings of young children's flexibility and locus of control predicted significantly mothers' parenting stress. In particular, when entered first, mothers' ratings of young children's flexibility predicted significantly mothers' parenting stress. When mothers' locus of control was added to this equation, however, only locus of control was a significant predictor of parenting stress. Thus, mothers' locus of control mediated the relationship between young children's flexibility and parenting stress. The mediational value of mothers' locus of control was confirmed with a significant Sobel Test ($z = 3.61, p < .001$).

When examining locus of control as a mediator in the relationship between young children's activity level and parenting stress, young children's activity level predicted significantly mothers' locus of control. Next, young children's activity level predicted significantly mothers' parenting stress. Then, collectively, mothers' ratings of young children's activity level and locus of control predicted significantly mothers' parenting stress. In particular, when entered first, young children's activity level predicted significantly parenting stress. When mothers' locus of control was added to this equation, however, only locus of control was a significant predictor of parenting stress. Thus, mothers' locus of control fully mediated the relationship between young children's activity level and parenting stress. The mediational value of mothers' locus of control was confirmed with a significant Sobel Test ($z = -2.73, p < .01$).

Finally, when examining locus of control as a mediator in the relationship between young children's quality of mood and parenting stress, young children's mood quality predicted significantly mothers' locus of control. Next, young children's mood quality predicted significantly mothers' parenting stress. Then, collectively, young children's mood quality and locus of control predicted significantly mothers' parenting stress. In particular, when entered first, mothers' ratings of young children's mood quality predicted significantly parenting stress. When mothers' locus of control was added to this equation, however, only locus of control was a significant predictor of parenting stress. Thus, mothers' locus of control fully mediated the relationship between young children's mood quality and parenting stress. The mediational value of mothers' locus of control was confirmed with a significant Sobel Test ($z = 2.45, p < .01$).

Table 4. Hierarchical regression analyses

Variables	*B*	SE *B*	*β*
Internalizing Behavior Problems			
Block 1. $F(3, 66) = 6.98, p < .001, R^2 = .21$			
Child Activity Level	.05	.21	.03
Child Flexibility	-1.40	.39	-.46**
Child Mood Quality	-.15	.38	-.05
Block 2. $F(5, 64) = 6.82, p < .001, R^2 = .30$			
Child Activity Level	-.03	.20	-.02
Child Flexibility	-1.27	.41	-.42**
Child Mood Quality	-.19	.36	-.06
Child Trait Rating	-.29	.09	-.36**
Parental Locus of Control	.07	.12	.08
Block 3. $F(6, 63) = 5.65, p < .001, R^2 = .29$			
Child Activity Level	-.04	.20	-.02
Child Flexibility	-1.26	.41	-.42**
Child Mood Quality	-.17	.36	-.06
Child Trait Rating	-.26	.11	-.33*
Parental Locus of Control	.10	.13	.11
Parenting Stress	.04	.09	.07
Externalizing Behavior Problems			
Block 1. $F(3, 66) = 5.67, p < .01, R^2 = .17$			
Child Activity Level	.59	.22	.31**
Child Flexibility	-.48	.42	-.15
Child Mood Quality	-.42	.40	-.13
Block 2. $F(5, 64) = 6.72, p < .001, R^2 = .29$			
Child Activity Level	.43	.21	.22*
Child Flexibility	.02	.42	.01
Child Mood Quality	-.41	.37	-.13
Child Trait Rating	-.23	.09	-.28*
Parental Locus of Control	-.21	.12	-.23
Block 3. $F(6, 63) = 5.53, p < .001, R^2 = .28$			
Child Activity Level	.42	.21	.22
Child Flexibility	.03	.43	.01
Child Mood Quality	-.40	.38	-.13
Child Trait Rating	-.22	.11	-.26*
Parental Locus of Control	-.19	.14	-.21
Parenting Stress	.27	.09	.05

Note. * $p < .05$; ** $p < .01$.

Predicting behavior problems

Finally, hierarchical regression analyses were used to determine the relative contributions of young children's temperament (i.e., greater activity level, flexibility, and mood quality) in Block 1, parents' attributions (i.e., child trait conceptions and locus of control attributions; controllability over parent-child interactions was not used as it was not related to young children's behavior problems) in Block 2, and parenting stress in Block 3 in predicting children's internalizing and externalizing behavior problems. Results of these analyses are in Table 4.

First, a hierarchical regression analysis examining young children's internalizing behavior problems showed that young children's flexibility contributed significantly to the prediction of young children's internalizing behavior problems in Block 1. In particular, a less flexible behavioral style was related to higher levels of young children's internalizing behavior problems. In Block 2, the regression equation remained significant when mothers' attributions were added. In this block, young children's flexibility and mothers' child trait conceptions served as significant predictors, with a less flexible behavioral style and less positive trait conceptions being related to higher levels of young children's internalizing behavior problems. In Block 3, the regression equation remained significant with the addition of parenting stress. Mothers' ratings of young children's flexibility and mothers' child trait conceptions served as significant predictors. Thus, less flexible behavioral style and less positive child trait conceptions were the strongest predictors of young children's internalizing behavior problems.

Next, a hierarchical regression analysis examining young children's externalizing behavior problems showed that young children's activity level contributed significantly to the prediction of externalizing behavior problems in Block 1. In particular, higher activity level was related to higher externalizing behavior problems. In Block 2, the regression equation remained significant with the addition of mothers' attributions. In this block, mothers' child trait conceptions were a significant predictor, with less positive trait attributions being related to higher levels of children's externalizing behavior problems. In Block 3, the regression equation remained significant with the addition of parenting stress. In this block, only mothers' child trait conceptions remained a significant predictor. Thus, negative child trait conceptions were the strongest predictor of young children's externalizing behavior problems.

DISCUSSION

The results of this study suggested that it is important to examine mothers' attributions as explanatory variables in the relationships between young children's temperament and mothers' parenting stress. Further, mothers' attributions proved to be important predictors of young children's behavior problems. Overall, the findings of this study suggested that mothers' child trait conceptions and locus of control mediate the relationship between their young children's temperament and their own parenting stress. Further, mothers' child trait conceptions and locus of control served as significant predictors of young children's behavior problems, even when young children's temperament and mothers' parenting stress also were entered into hierarchical regression equations. Although mothers' attributions were important, different attributions demonstrated unique patterns of results.

In particular, mothers' ratings of their young children's activity level and lower flexibility were related positively and significantly to less positive child trait conceptions. Consistent with previous research, this finding may suggest that attributions become schematic and promote automatic influences on the perception and subsequent processing of young children's behavior (50). Thus, parents who hold more negative child trait conceptions may be more likely to automatically perceive their young children's temperament as difficult. Contrary to expectations, however, the quality of young children's mood was unrelated to mothers' child trait conceptions, possibly due to young children's mood being viewed as a more transient characteristic (i.e., as opposed to a fixed characteristic) of young children's temperament.

In addition, this study demonstrated that mothers' ratings of young children's flexibility and quality of mood are related significantly and positively to mothers' locus of control. In contrast, mothers' ratings of children's activity level were related significantly and negatively to mothers' locus of control. These findings were consistent with previous research (12), which suggested that the interactions between mothers and their children who have difficult temperaments are based on trying to relieve children's distress and are likely to be unsuccessful. Accordingly, due to unsuccessful attempts at trying to relieve children's distress, mothers of children who have difficult temperaments may believe that they have no control over their children's behavior. As a result, these mother-child pairs may benefit from added intervention targeting mothers' attributions and young children's behavior problems.

Finally, contrary to previous literature (50), parents' attributions of controllability over parent-child interactions were unrelated to the other variables examined in this study. This lack of relationships may be a result of the sample used in the present study. Specifically, the participants in the current study were considerably different from the participant sample used to validate the PAT (i.e., parents in the current study were higher in socioeconomic status and had children who were not experiencing clinically concerning difficulties) (50). Accordingly, the range of ratings provided by the parents in the current study may not be broad enough to produce statistically significant results. Future research should examine the potential differences in parents' ratings of controllability over parent-child interactions in the context of interactions between diverse parents and their children.

With regard to the experience of parenting stress, mothers who reported that their young children displayed more difficult temperament characteristics also reported higher parenting stress. In addition, mothers who reported more negative child trait conceptions and an external locus of control endorsed higher parenting stress. Overall, these findings were similar to those of previous research (30). An alternate explanation of these findings may be, however, that parenting stress may prompt parents to perceive their young children as having less favorable child traits and to believe that they have less control in interactions with their young children. Because the design of this study did not allow for the directionality of these relationships to be determined, these relationships deserve further study.

With regard to the question of attributions as mediators, this study demonstrated that mothers' child trait conceptions fully mediated the relationship between young children's activity level and mothers' parenting stress and partially mediated the relationship between young children's flexibility and mothers' parenting stress. Consistent with previous literature, parents who make positive child trait conceptions may be more likely to help their children overcome problems and to contribute to positive developmental outcomes (51). Further, more negative child trait conceptions may be related to negative interpretations of and responses to children's behaviors (19) and to increases in parenting stress (31). Further, locus of control served as a mediator as well, with young children's temperament predicting mothers' locus of control attributions and these attributions predicting mothers' ratings of their parenting stress. Thus, mothers' attributions of their ability to influence their young children's behavior may have significant value when attempting to understand the relationship between young children's temperament and mothers' parenting stress. Such information may suggest that helping mothers to alter their child trait conceptions and their locus of control as part of parenting interventions may prove useful in promoting less parenting stress and more positive young child outcomes.

Overall, these results lend support to the idea of 'harmonious parenting.' In particular, the concept of harmonious parenting describes parents who are able to successfully adapt to the needs of their children and effectively influence their children's behavior. As a result, these parents were more likely to have children who were attached securely and were better able to cope effectively with their emotional responses and distress (11). Thus, if parents are able to attribute their young children's behavior to temperament, they may better adapt their parenting to fit the needs of their young children, to decrease their parenting stress, and to increase the likelihood of a 'good fit' with their young children. Thus, it may be that parents' contribution to the parent-child relationship is dependent on young children's temperament and parents' attributions.

This study also examined the relative contributions of young children's temperament, mothers' attributions, and mothers' parenting stress in predicting young children's behavior problems. When examining young children's behavior problems, the majority of the variables in this study were related significantly to young children's behavior problems. These findings were consistent with previous research that suggested that children's difficult temperament (8), parents' negative attributions (22, 40), and parents' increased levels of parenting stress (31) were associated individually with children's behavior problems. When examined together in the context of hierarchical regression analyses, however, only mothers' ratings of their young children's flexibility and their child trait conceptions contributed significantly to young children's internalizing behavior problems. For young children's externalizing behavior problems, only mothers' child trait conceptions served as a significant predictor. Thus, mothers who reported that their young children had a more rigid behavioral style and who endorsed less positive child trait conceptions were more likely to endorse that their young children were exhibiting higher levels of behavior problems. These findings were actually somewhat surprising, as the extant literature suggested that temperament and later psychological symptoms consisted of overlapping behavioral indicators and demonstrated significant relationships (e.g., 52). Nonetheless, the results of this study suggested that young children's temperament may be related to mothers' attributions and the way in which mothers think and behave toward their young children (40). Such findings would suggest that improving mothers' ability to reflect on their perceptions of themselves and of their children may be an important component to successful parenting interventions. This hypothesis should be examined in future research.

Given these findings, it will be important for researchers and health service providers to collect information from multiple informants when assessing young children's behavior problems. Such cross-informant information may improve the understanding of young children's behavior problems, especially since different informants may hold different attributions regarding young children's behavior. Further, the findings of this study suggested that parenting interventions should include a component that addresses parents' attributions of their young children's temperament, their reflective functioning, and the role that they believe they play in parenting interactions with their young children. Such changes in attributions may increase the likelihood of parents and their children experiencing a 'good fit,' regardless of young children's temperament.

The results of this study should be viewed within the context of its limitations. First, although the number of participating mothers in this study was adequate, not enough fathers provided information for meaningful data analyses to be conducted. Further, there were a considerable number of parents who did not return their research packets despite consenting to participate. Thus, participating mothers may not be representative of the general population. Specifically, these mothers were among a select group of parents who participated despite not receiving compensation for their participation, who were mostly Caucasian, and whose children were enrolled in private preschools. These demographic characteristics may have been related to the results of this study and their generalizability. Further, this study relied solely on mothers' self-reports. As a result, mothers' ratings may not reflect their own or their children's actual behavior. Finally, from a methodological perspective, some researchers feel that mediation only can be tested in the context of longitudinal relationships, which was not possible in the current study.

Despite the limitations of this study, the findings reported here emphasized the importance of mothers' attributions, particularly when examining the relationships among young children's temperament, mothers' parenting stress, and young children's behavior problems. In this study, mothers' child trait conceptions fully mediated the relationship between young children's activity level and parenting stress and partially mediated the relationship between young children's flexibility and parenting stress. In addition, mothers' locus of control attributions fully mediated the relationship between all three temperament dimensions (i.e., activity level, flexibility, and quality of mood) and parenting stress. When examined together in hierarchical regression analyses, mothers' ratings of their young children's flexibility and child trait conceptions contributed significantly to mothers' ratings of young children's internalizing behavior problems. Further, when examined in hierarchical regression analyses, mothers' child trait conceptions contributed significantly to mothers' ratings of young children's externalizing behavior problems. Future research would benefit from studying the directionality of the relationships found among the variables in this study and from examining a more diverse population. In addition, future research would benefit from examining the role that fathers' attributions play in the relationship between young children's temperament, parenting stress, and young children's behavior problems, as fathers' attributions may have differential relationships. Overall, parenting interventions would benefit from targeting mothers' attributions of their young children in conjunction with addressing young children's behavior problems and mothers' parenting stress.

REFERENCES

[1] Calkins SD, Hungerford A, Dedmon SE. Mothers' interactions with temperamentally frustrated infants. Inf Ment Health J 2004;25:219-39.

[2] Bugental DB, Blue J, Cruzcosa M. Perceived control over caregiving outcomes: Implications for child abuse. Dev Psychol 1989;25:631-8.

[3] Deater-Deckard K. Parenting stress and children's development: Introduction to the special issue. Inf Child Dev 2005;14:111-5.

[4] Rubin KH, Burgess KB, Dwyer KM, Hastings PD. Predicting preschoolers' externalizing behaviors from toddler temperament, conflict, and maternal negativity. Dev Psychol 2003;39:164-76.

[5] Rothbart MK, Bates JE. Temperament. In: Damon W, Eisenberg N, eds. Handbook of child psychology. Vol 3: Social, emotional and personality development, Sixth edition. New York: Wiley, 2006:99-166.

[6] Bates JE, Maslin CA, Frankel KA. Attachment security, mother-child interaction, and temperament as predictors of behavior problem ratings at age three years. Soc Res Child Dev 1985;50(1-2):167-93.

[7] van den Akker AL, Dekovic´ M, Prinzie P, Asscher JJ. Toddlers' temperament profiles: Stability and relations to negative and positive parenting. J Abnorm Child Psychol 2010;38:485-95.

[8] Thomas A, Chess S, Birch HG. Temperament and behavior disorders in children. New York: New York University Press, 1968.

[9] Billman J, McDevitt SC. Convergence of parent and observer ratings of temperament with observations of peer interaction in nursery school. Child Dev 1980;51:395-400.

[10] Windle M, Lerner RM. Reassessing the dimensions of temperamental individuality across the life span: The revised dimensions of temperament survey (DOTS-R). J Adolesc Res 1986;1:213–30.

[11] Bowlby J. Attachment and loss. Vol 1: Attachment (2nd edition). New York: Basic Books, 1982.

[12] Van den Boom DC, Hoeksma JB. The effect of infant irritability on mother-infant interaction: A growth-curve analysis. Dev Psychol 1994;30:581-90.

[13] Murray L, Stanley C, Hooper R, King F, Fiori-Cowley A. The role of infant factors in postnatal depression and mother-infant interactions. Dev Med Child Neurol 1996;38:109-19.

[14] Smith AM, O'Leary SG. Attributions and arousal as predictors of maternal discipline. Cog Ther Res 1995;19:459-71.

[15] Bryan A, Dix T. Mothers' emotions and behavioral support during interactions with toddlers: The role of child temperament. Soc Dev 2009;18:647-70.

[16] Miller SA. Parents' attributions for their children's behavior. Child Dev 1995;66:1557-84.

[17] Weiner B. An attributional theory of motivation and emotion. New York: Springer, 1986.

[18] Bugental DB, Johnston C. Parental and child cognitions in the context of the family. Annu Rev Psychol 2000;51:315-44.

[19] Sacco WP, Murray DW. Mother-child relationship satisfaction: The role of attributions and trait conceptions. J Soc Clin Psychol 1997;16:24-42.

[20] Carlston DE, Skowronski JJ. Savings in the learning of trait information as evidence for spontaneous inference generation. J Pers Soc Psychol 1994;66:840-56.

[21] Rotter JB. Generalized expectancies for internal versus external control of reinforcement. Psychol Monogr 1966;80 (1):1-28.

[22] Bugental DB, Shennum WA. "Difficult" children as elicitors and targets of adult communication patterns: An attributional behavioral transactional analysis. Monogr Soc Res Child Dev 1984;49:1-70.

[23] Bugental DB, Caporael L, Shennum WA. Experimentally produced child uncontrollability over parent-child interactions: Effects on the potency of adult communication patterns. Child Dev 1980;51:520-8.

[24] Carton JS, Carton ER. Nonverbal maternal warmth and children's locus of control of reinforcement. J Nonverbal Behav 2008;22:77-86.

[25] Dix T, Grusec J. Parent attribution processes in the socialization of children. In: Sigel IE, ed. Parental belief systems. Hillsdale, NJ: Erlbaum, 1985:201-33.

[26] Patterson GR. Coercive family process. Eugene, OR: Castalia, 1982.

[27] Rubin KH, Mills RSL. Maternal beliefs about adaptive and maladaptive social behaviors in normal, aggressive, and withdrawn preschoolers. J Abnorm Child Psychol 1990;18:419-35.

[28] Esdaile SA, Greenwood KM. A comparison of mothers' and fathers' experience of parenting stress and attributions for parent-child interaction outcomes. Occup Ther Int 2003;10:115-26.

[29] Abidin RR. Parenting stress index (PSI) manual. Odessa, FL: Psychological Assessment Resources, 1990.

[30] Abidin RR. Parenting stress index: Professional manual, 3rd ed. New York: Psychological Assessment Resources, 1995.

[31] Creasey GL, Jarvis PA. Relationships between parenting stress and developmental functioning among 2-year-olds. Inf Behav Dev 1994;17:423-9.

[32] Fischer M. Parenting stress and the child with attention deficit hyperactivity disorder. J Clin Child Psychol 1990;19:337-46.

[33] Jouriles EN, Murphy CM, O'Leary KD. Effects of maternal mood on mother-son interaction patterns. J Abnorm Child Psychol 1989;17:513-25.

[34] Lahey BB, Conger R, Atkeson BM, Treiber FA. Parenting behavior and emotional status of physically abusive mothers. J Consult Clin Psychol 1984;52:252-6.

[35] Eisenberg N, Cumberland A, Sprinrad TL, Fabes RA, Shepard SA, Reiser M. The relations of regulation and emotionality to children's externalizing and internalizing problem behavior. Child Dev 2001;71:1112-34.

[36] Campbell SB, Shaw DS, Gilliom, M. Early externalizing behavior problems: Toddlers and preschoolers at risk for later maladjustment. Dev Psychopath 2000;12:467-88.

[37] Denham SA, Workman E, Cole PM, Weissbrod C, Kendziora KT, Zhan-Waxler C. Predictions of externalizing behavior problems from early to middle childhood: The role of parental socialization and emotion expression. Dev Psychopath 2000;12: 23-45.

[38] Eisenberg N, Valiente C, Spinrad TL, Cumberland A, Liew J, Reiser M, et al. Longitudinal relations to children's effortful control, impulsivity, and negative emotionality to their externalizing, internalizing, and co-occurring behavior problems. Dev Psychol 2009;45:988-1008.

[39] Karreman A, de Haas S, van Tuijl C, van Aken MAG, Dekovic´ M. Relations among temperament, parenting and problem behavior in young children. Inf Behav Dev 2010;33:39-49.

[40] Strassberg Z. Social information processing in compliance situations by mothers of behavior-problem boys. Child Dev 1995;66:376-89.

[41] Cohen J. A power primer. Psychol Bull 1992;112:155-9.

[42] Sacco WP, Johnson SA, Tenzer SA. Parent perceptions, affective reactions, and depression in children. Paper presented at the 101st Annual Convention of the American Psychological Association, Toronto, Canada, August 1993.

[43] Rayfield A, Eyberg SM, Boggs S, Roberts M. Parenting locus of control: Short form. November 1995. URL: http://www.phhp.ufl.edu/~eyberg/NewTemplateFolder/Measures.htm.

[44] Campis LK, Lyman RD, Prentice-Dunn S. The parental locus of control scale: Development and validation. J Clin Child Psychol 1986;15:260-7.

[45] Rayfield A, Eyberg SM, Boggs S, Roberts M. Development and validation of the Parenting Locus of Control-Short Form. Paper presented at the annual meeting of the AABT Preconference on Social Learning and the Family, Washington, DC, November 1995.

[46] Bugental DB. Parent attribution test (Manual). [On-Line], 1998. URL: http://www.psych.ucsb.edu/~bugental/pat.english.doc.

[47] Achenbach TM, Rescorla LA. Manual for the ASEBA preschool forms and profiles. Burlington, VT: University Vermont Department Psychiatry, 2000.

[48] Achenbach TM, Rescorla LA. Manual for the ASEBA school-age forms and profiles. Burlington, VT: University of Vermont Research Center for Children Youth Families, 2001.

[49] Baron RM, Kenny DA. The moderator-mediator variable distinction in social psychological research: Conceptual, strategic, and statistical considerations. J Pers Soc Psychol 1986;51:1173-82.

[50] Bugental DB. Affective and cognitive processes within threat-oriented family systems. In: Sigel IE, McGillicuddy-DeLisi AV, Goodnow JJ, eds. Parental belief systems, 2nd edition. Hillsdale, NJ: Earlbaum, 1992:219-48.

[51] Gretarsson SJ, Gelfand DM. Mother's attributions regarding their children's social behavior and personality characteristics. Dev Psychol 1988;24:264-9.

[52] Frick PJ. Integrating research on temperament and childhood psychopathology: Its pitfalls and promise. J Clin Child Adolesc Psychol 2004;33:2-7.

In: Childhood and Adolescence
Editor: Joav Merrick

ISBN: 978-1-53613-574-9

Chapter 9

Does Head and Neck Cancer (HNC) Education Have an Impact on Adolescents' Knowledge and Attitude Towards HNC and HNC Peer Education? An Example from Nigeria

Kehinde K Kanmodi[1,2,3], BDS
and Omotayo F Fagbule[1,4], BDS, MWACS
[1]Campaign for Head and Neck Cancer Education Program,
Cephas Health Research Initiative Inc, Ibadan, Nigeria
[2]Department of Dental and Maxillofacial Surgery,
Usmanu Danfodiyo University Teaching Hospital, Sokoto, Nigeria
[3]Community Health Officers Training Programme,
Usmanu Danfodiyo University Teaching Hospital, Sokoto, Nigeria
[4]Department of Periodontology and Community Dentistry,
University College Hospital, Ibadan, Nigeria

Health education has been found effective in reducing the prevalence of risky pro-cancer behaviors among adolescents. For this reason, the

Cephas Health Research Initiative Inc, Nigeria, embarked on the CHANCE (Campaign for Head and Neck Cancer Education) Program to reduce the prevalence of head and neck cancer (HNC) risk factors among Nigerian adolescents. *Objectives:* To explore the impact of HNC education on secondary school students' knowledge of the etiologies and symptoms of head and neck cancer (HNC). To also explore the impact of HNC education on their willingness to educate their peers about HNC. Materials and Methods: An interventional study was conducted among grades 10 to 12 students (n = 103) in a public high school in Ilesa Town, Southwestern Nigeria. A well-structured questionnaire was used to obtain information from each participant before and after a session of HNC education. Collected data were cleaned, and analyzed using SPSS version 16 software. *Results:* The mean age (±SD) of respondents was 13.89 (±1.01) years, 72.8% were males, while 82.5% were Yorubas. There was a remarkable increase in the mean (±SD) knowledge scores of respondents' knowledge of HNC etiology/risk factors (7.3% [±22.5%] versus 68.3% [±32.4%]) and symptoms (9.1% [±23.9%] versus 71.4% [±33.3%]) after the session of HNC education. There was a statistically significant increase in the number of respondents that were willing to educate their friends about HNC cancer after the education session (87.4% [pre-test] versus 88.3% [post-test], [X^2: p < 0.001; df = 4]). *Conclusion*: Head and neck cancer education markedly improved the subjects' knowledge of HNC. Adolescents can be made peer educators on HNC if made knowledgeable about the disease.

INTRODUCTION

Head and neck cancer (HNC) is a killer disease (1). Globally, more than 55,000 newly diagnosed cases and around 300,000 HNC-associated deaths are recorded yearly (1). Some of the most popular risk factors associated with HNC include tobacco, alcohol, and human papillomavirus (2-4).

The global prevalence of HNC risk factors among adolescents is alarming (5-7). In a developing country like Nigeria, the prevalence rates of HNC risk factors like tobacco use, oral sex, and alcoholism has been recorded to be >10% among different populations of surveyed adolescents (8-15). This suggests the need for an effective health promotion program that is focused on HNC disease prevention among Nigerian adolescents.

A sound knowledge of diseases is very important in health promotion and disease prevention (16). If an individual is made knowledgeable about a disease, he/she will be able to take preventive measures against having such disease (17). In the quest for promoting healthy practices among Nigerians, a non-profit non-governmental organization called "Cephas Health Research Initiative Inc" was founded in the year 2016 (18). This organization was established with the purpose of reducing the prevalence of diseases in Nigeria through health advocacy and health research. This organization, in December, 2016, launched the community-based health promotion program called "Campaign for Head and Neck Cancer Education (CHANCE)" with the aim of educating people on HNC disease.

For this charity organization to effectively carry out her educational programs on HNC, it is very important for her to conduct scientific research to evaluate the impact of these programs. The findings made from such research will definitely provide this organization with vital information on the areas that need to be strengthened in her educational programs.

Based on the above, the HNC educators of this charity organization aimed to conduct this study to evaluate the impact of this organization's first HNC school education program on the: 1) knowledge and attitude of some Nigerian adolescents on HNC; 2) and their attitude towards HNC peer education.

OUR STUDY

This research was an interventional study conducted during a school outreach program which held at a public high school in Ilesa Town, Nigeria, on December 2, 2016. This study was conducted under the guidelines of the Helsinki Declaration on health research. Approval to conduct this study was officially obtained from the school authority. Also, all subject's participation was strictly confidential and voluntary.

It was announced, by the school authority, during the early hours of the day of this outreach program that those students in Grades 10 to 12 will be given a health talk. About three hours after the end of the academic activities for the day, a total of 187 Grades 10 to 12 students who were interested in the health talk were assembled in the school auditorium for the program.

The study instrument was an anonymous pretest-posttest questionnaire developed from the HNC information obtained from the webpage of the American Academy of Otolaryngology – Head and Neck Surgery (19). Both the pretest and the posttest questionnaires obtained information from the participants about their bio-data, knowledge of the etiology/risk factors and symptoms of HNC, as well their attitudes towards educating their peers on HNC. In the posttest questionnaire, the participants were further asked if they enjoyed the HNC education program; this question was asked to check if the program was interesting to the students.

Before the health talk, a total of 103 randomly selected consenting subjects (out of the 187 students that attended the program) were given a pre-test questionnaire to fill and return. Thereafter, a 45-minute health talk on HNC was delivered to the students by a dental surgeon (KKK). During the health talk, the meaning of HNC, HNC etiology/risk factors, HNC symptoms, and HNC self-examination were clearly explained to the participants using simple and comprehensible terms. After the health talk, the participating students were requested to ask questions. Another 15 minutes was devoted to answer all questions relevant to the scope of the health talk. After the question and answer session, the pre-tested 103 students were issued the posttest questionnaires to fill and return.

No questionnaire was discarded because they were all properly filled. The statistical tool used for the data analysis was the SPSS version 16 Software. Before the data coding and entry into the SPSS, the subjects' pretest and posttest responses to the etiology/risk factors and symptoms of HNC were marked and scored over 100. Thereafter, all data (including the knowledge scores of the subjects on the etiology/risk factors and symptoms of HNC) were coded and entered into the SPSS version 16 Software. The frequency distribution of all variables were determined, and comparison between variables were also done using the Chi-square test, with a p-value of <0.05 set to establish the level of statistical significance. The results generated were presented using tables and chart.

FINDINGS

The mean age (±SD) of the 103 subjects was 13.89 (±1.01) years, 72.8% were males, 82.5% were Yorubas, 76.7% were Christians, and 95.1% were boarding students (see Table 1). The majority (70.0%) of the subjects were also in their 10th grade (see Figure 2). There was a remarkable increase in the subjects' mean (±SD) knowledge scores on HNC etiology/risk factors (7.3% [±22.5%] versus 68.3% [±32.4%]) and symptoms (9.1% [±23.9%] versus 71.4% [±33.3%]) after the session of HNC education (see Table 2).

It was also observed that there was a statistically significant increase in the number of subjects that were willing to educate their friends about HNC cancer after the education session (87.4% [pre-test] versus 88.3% [post-test], [X^2: $p < 0.001$; $df = 4$]) (see Table 3).

Lastly, the majority (92.2%) of the subjects enjoyed the HNC education program (see Table 4).

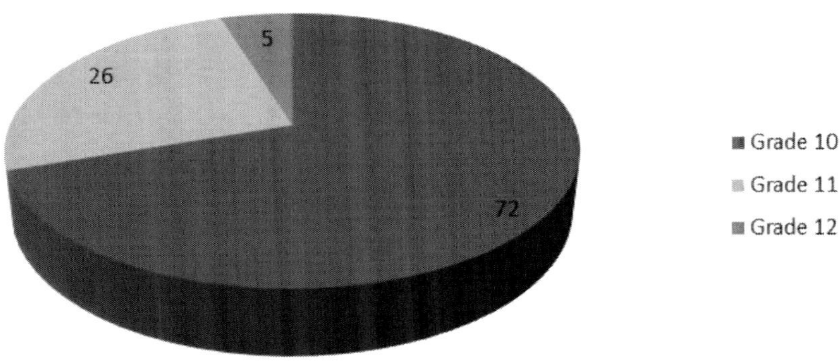

Figure 1. Frequency distribution of the school grades of the subjects.

Table 1. Demographic profile of the subjects

Characteristics (n = 103)	Frequency (%)
Gender	
Male	75 (72.8)
Female	24 (23.3)
Not specified	4 (3.9)
Mean age* (±SD)	13.89 (±1.01)
Tribe	
Yoruba	85 (82.5)
Hausa	2 (1.9)
Igbo	13 (12.6)
Others	3 (2.9)
Religion	
Christian	79 (76.7)
Islam	23 (22.3)
Others	1 (1.0)
Mode of studentship	
Day student	4 (3.9)
Boarding student	98 (95.1)
Not specified	1 (1.0)

*Age was recorded in years.

Table 2. Knowledge scores of the subjects before and after the session of HNC health education program

Variables	P_0 (±SD)	P_1 (±SD)	$P_1 - P_0$
Knowledge of etiology of HNC*	7.3 (±22.5)	68.3 (±32.4)	61.0
Knowledge of symptoms of HNC*	9.1 (±23.9)	71.4 (±33.3)	62.3

*Knowledge of all the respondents was measured using mean scores (all values were recorded in percentages); SD = Standard deviation; P_1 = Posttest; P_0 = Pretest; $P_1 - P_0$ = Increase in the respondents' mean knowledge scores after the intervention.

Table 3. Impact of HNC education on the attitude of the subjects toward HNC peer education

Question	Now that you have been educated on how to prevent HNC, will you be willing to educate your friends about HNC?*					p-value
If you are educated on how to prevent HNC, will you be willing to teach your friends about it?*		Yes	No	NS	Total	
	Yes	90	0	0	90	<0.0001
	No	1	1	0	2	
	NS	0	0	0	1	
	Total	91	1	1	93	

*Only 10 subjects gave incomplete responses to the cross-tabulated questions; hence their data were not computed in this statistics; NS = Not sure.

Table 4. Response of the subjects to the question: Did you enjoy the HNC education you just received?

Response	Frequency (%)
Yes	95 (92.2)
No	1 (1.0)
Indifferent	2 (1.9)
No response	5 (4.9)
Total	103 (100.0)

Discussion

Health education is an effective tool for disease prevention (16). Health education, according to the World Health Organization, can be defined as any combination of learning experience designed to help individuals and communities improve their health, by increasing their knowledge or influencing their attitudes (17). Health education has been found effective in reducing the prevalence of disease risk factors in different countries of the world (16, 20, 21).

In this study, the impact of HNC education on the knowledge and attitudes of high school adolescents on HNC disease and HNC peer education was positive. This study showed that school HNC education program is an effective tool in creating awareness on HNC. This study also showed that school HNC education program is interesting to adolescents, and many of them are willing to be peer educators on HNC if made knowledgeable about the disease.

Authors would like to recommend that school HNC education programs should be embraced by health educators in creating awareness on the risk factors, symptoms, and self-screening of HNC among adolescents.

ACKNOWLEDGMENTS

This study was funded by the authors. The opinions expressed in this paper are that of the authors and not necessarily of the organizations they are affiliated to. The authors deeply appreciate the Multinational Association for Supportive Care in Cancer (MASCC), Canada, for partly funding the trip for the poster presentation of this research at the 2017 MASCC/ISOO conference which held in Washington DC, USA, in June 2017 (22).

REFERENCES

[1] Jemal A, Bray F, Center MM, Ferlay J, Ward E, Forman D. Global cancer statistics. CA Cancer J Clin 2011;61(2):69-90.

[2] Shaw R, Beasley N. Aetiology and risk factors for head and neck cancer: United Kingdom National Multidisciplinary Guidelines. J Laryngol Otol 2016;130(Suppl 2):S9-S12.

[3] Singh J, Ramamoorthi R, Baxi S, Jayaraj R, Thomas M. The risk factors of head and neck cancer and their general patterns in Australia: A descriptive review and update. J Environ Pathol Toxicol Oncol 2014;33(1):45-7.

[4] Ragin CC, Modugno F, Gollin SM. The epidemiology and risk factors of head and neck cancer: a focus on human papillomavirus. J Dent Res 2007;86(2):104-114.

[5] Ng M, Freeman MK, Fleming TD, Robinson M, Dwyer-Lindgren L, et al. Smoking prevalence and cigarette consumption in 187 countries, 1980-2012. JAMA 2014;311(2):183-92.

[6] Xi B, Liang Y, Liu Y, Yan Y, Zhao M, Ma C, Bovet P. Tobacco use and second-hand smoke exposure in young adolescents aged 12-15 years: data from 68 low-income and middle-income countries. Lancet Glob Health 2016;4:e759-805.

[7] World Health Organization. Global status report on alcohol and health, 2011. Geneva: WHO, 2011.

[8] Odey FA, Okokon IB, Ogbeche JO, Jombo GT, Ekanem EE. Prevalence of cigarette smoking among adolescents in Calabar city, south-eastern Nigeria. J Med Sci 2012;3(4):237-42.

[9] Raji MO, Muhammad H, Usman AM, Umar M, Oladigbolu RA, Kaoje AU. Cigarette smoking among out-of-school adolescents in Sokoto metropolis, North-west Nigeria. Health Sci J 2017;11:3.

[10] Ebirim CIC, Amadi AN, Abanobi OC, Iloh GUC. The prevalence of cigarette smoking and knowledge of its health implications among adolescents in Owerri, South-Eastern Nigeria. Health 2014;6:1532-8.

[11] Adje DEU, Oyita GI, Eniojukan JF. Substance abuse among adolescents: prevalence and patterns of alcohol consumption among senior secondary school students in Abraka, Delta State, Nigeria. Sch Acad J Pharm 2015;4(1):63-9.

[12] Alex-Hart BA, Opara PI, Okagua J. Prevalence of alcohol consumption among secondary school students in Port Harcourt, Southern Nigeria. Niger J Paed 2015;42(1):39-45.

[13] Afolabi MO, Ayilara AE, Akinyemi OA, Ola-Olorun OJ. Survey of drug use among young people in Ife, Nigeria. Afr J Drug Alcohol Stud 2012;11(2):87-94.

[14] Bamidele JO, Abodunrin OL, Adebimpe WO. Sexual behaviours and risk of HIV/AIDS among adolescents in public secondary schools in Osogbo, Osun State, Nigeria. Int J Adolesc Med Health 2009;21(3):387-94.

[15] Famutimi EO, Oyetunde MO. Risky sexual behavior among secondary school adolescents in Ibadan North Local Government Area, Nigeria. J Nursing Health Sci 2014;3(3):34-44.

[16] Pawloski ZS, Gromadecka-Sutiewicz M, Skommer J, Paul M, et al. Impact of health education on knowledge and prevention behavior for congenital toxoplasmosis: the experience in Poznan, Poland. Health Educ Res 2001;16(4):493-502.

[17] World Health Organization. Health education. URL: www.who.int/topics/health_education/en/.

[18] Cephas Health Research Initiative. Mission. URL: www.chrinitiative.org/about-us/mission/.

[19] American Academy of Otolaryngology. Head and neck cancer. URL: www.entnet.org/content/head-and-neck-cancer.

[20] Briegger WR, Adeniyi JD, Parker KA, Oldepo O. Health education in Africa: 1975-2000. Health Educ Res 2000;15(4):383-91.

[21] Albert C, Davia M. Education is a key determinant of health in Europe: A comparative analysis of 11 countries. Health Prom Int 2010;26(2):163-70.

[22] Kanmodi K, Fagbule F. Impact of head and neck cancer (HNC) education on Nigerian adolescents' knowledge and attitudes towards HNC and HNC education advocacy: the CHANCE* Pilot Study. Support Care Cancer 2017;25(Suppl 1):S168.

In: Childhood and Adolescence
Editor: Joav Merrick
ISBN: 978-1-53613-574-9

Chapter 10

SECONDHAND TOBACCO SMOKE EXPOSURE AND ATTITUDES TOWARDS THE TOBACCO BAN: A PILOT SURVEY OF SECONDARY SCHOOL STUDENTS IN IBOKUN TOWN, NIGERIA

Omotayo F Fagbule*[1,2]*, BDS, MWACS,
Kehinde K Kanmodi*[1,3,4,*]*, BDS
and Timothy O Aladelusi*[1,5,6,7]*, BDS, MSc, FWACS, FAOCMF

[1]Campaign for Head and Neck Cancer Education (CHANCE) Program, Cephas Health Research Initiative Inc, Ibadan, Nigeria
[2]Department of Periodontology and Community Dentistry, University College Hospital, Ibadan, Nigeria
[3]Department of Dental and Maxillofacial Surgery, Usmanu Danfodiyo University Teaching Hospital, Sokoto, Nigeria

[*] Correspondence: Kehinde K Kanmodi, BDS, Cephas Health Research Initiative Inc, Ibadan, Nigeria. Email: kanmodikehinde@yahoo.com.

[4]Community Health Officers Training Programme,
Usmanu Danfodiyo University Teaching Hospital, Sokoto, Nigeria
[5]Department of Oral and Maxillofacial Surgery,
University of Ibadan, Ibadan, Nigeria
[6]Department of Oral and Maxillofacial Surgery,
University College Hospital, Ibadan, Nigeria
[7]Ninth People's Hospital, Shanghai, Peoples Republic of China

Secondhand tobacco smoke continues to be responsible for the deaths of many people yearly. Objectives: To explore the prevalence of recent exposure to secondhand tobacco smoke. Methods: A cross-section of 198 Grades 10 to 12 students from two conveniently selected secondary schools in Ibokun, Nigeria, was surveyed in this questionnaire-based study. Information on biodata, exposure to secondhand tobacco smokes, school's enforcement of tobacco ban policy, and attitudes towards ban of public advertisement, sales and smoking of tobacco were obtained from each participant. Data collected was analyzed using the SPSS version 16 Software. Results: More than half (54.0%) of the respondents were 14 years old, 56.6% of them were females, 82.8% were in grades 10 to 12, 50.5% were in a private school. Only nine respondents had been exposed to secondhand tobacco smokes daily, both at places within and outside their residential areas, within the recent seven days prior to the day of participation in this study. A higher proportion of those respondents from private school, when compared to those from public school, reported that tobacco ban policy is enforced in their school. Also, a higher proportion of the males, when compared to the females supported a ban on the sales, advertisements, smoking of tobacco in public places. Conclusion: In this survey, only a few students were recently exposed to secondhand tobacco smoke. The majority of them support the ban of advertisements, sales, and use of tobacco and tobacco products in public places.

INTRODUCTION

Exposure to secondhand tobacco smoke continues to be a major problem of global health concern (1, 2). According to the World Health Organization, second-hand tobacco smoke is responsible for the deaths of about 600,000 people yearly, and more than 70% of these deaths occur in low-income and middle-income countries like Nigeria (1).

In May 2015, the Federal Government of Nigeria passed the tobacco control bill into law, prohibiting smoking in public places (3, 4). The public places where smoking is prohibited in the Nigerian law include schools, healthcare centers, amusement parks, stadia, restaurants, public transportation parks, gardens and plazas.

Studies had shown that about 14.5-55.8% of secondary school students in the major Nigerian cities are exposed to secondhand tobacco smokes, both at home and at public places (4, 5). After extensive literature search, the authors observed that only scanty studies were available on secondhand tobacco smoke exposure among secondary school students in the semi-urban and rural areas in Nigeria. Based on this, the authors aimed to conduct a pilot study to determine the rate of exposure to secondhand tobacco smokes among secondary school students in two secondary schools in Ibokun Town (Ibokun is a semi-urban town in Nigeria), and also explore their attitudes towards ban on advertisement, sales and use of tobacco in public places. This study is of high significance, as it gives an insight on the rate of secondhand tobacco exposure among secondary school students in Ibokun, and also explores their attitude towards tobacco ban policy.

OUR STUDY

This study was a cross-sectional pilot study conducted under the guidelines of the Helsinki Declaration on health research involving human subjects. Prior to the study, authors obtained permission to carry out the study from the authorities of the participating schools. Informed verbal consent was also obtained from the school teachers and study participants after clearly explaining the aims and objectives of the study to the teachers and participants. All participation was voluntary and anonymous.

The study was carried out among grades 10 to 12 students from two conveniently selected secondary schools (one private and one public) in Ibokun Town, Osun State, Nigeria. Ibokun is a semi-urban area in Osun State, and the occupation of the inhabitants is predominantly farming (6).

The study instrument used for this study was an anonymous questionnaire developed from literatures (4, 5). The questionnaire obtained information from each participant on their biodata, exposure to secondhand tobacco smoke, enforcement of tobacco ban policy in their school, and attitudes towards public advertisement, sales and use of tobacco products.

A convenient sample of 198 Grades 10 to 12 students from two conveniently selected secondary schools in Ibokun, Nigeria, was surveyed in this study. Multistage sampling technique was used in the selection of the participating classes, thereafter simple random sampling technique was adopted in the selection of participants from the selected classes. Data for this study was collected in the months of November and December, 2016.

Data cleaning was done and no questionnaire was found worthy of being discarded because all were properly filled. Data was entered into the SPSS version 16 Software for analysis. Frequency distributions of all variables were determined, and comparisons between variables were also done using the Chi-square test; a p-value of <0.005 was set to be the level of statistical significance. The outcomes of the analysis were presented using tables.

FINDINGS

More than half (54.0%) of the respondents were $\leq$14 years old, 56.6% of them were females, 82.8% were in grades 10 to 12, 50.5% were in a private school, 97.5% were Yorubas, and 74.2% were Christians (see Table 1).

Only nine respondents had been exposed to secondhand tobacco smokes, both at places within and outside their residential areas, on all the seven days prior to the day of participation in this study. Overall, more females were exposed to secondhand tobacco smokes within the recent seven days prior to the day of participation in this study, when compared to the males (see Tables 2 and 3).

Table 1. Demographic profile of respondents

Characteristics (n=198)	Frequency (%)
Gender	
Female	112 (56.6)
Male	81 (40.9)
Not specified	5 (2.5)
School grade	
Grades 7 – 9	37 (17.2)
Grades 10 – 12	161 (82.8)
Age (in years)	
≤14	107 (54.0)
15 – 18	83 (41.9)
19 – 24	3 (1.5)
Not specified	5 (2.5)
School	
Public	98 (49.5)
Private	100 (50.5)
Tribe	
Yoruba	193 (97.5)
Igbo	1 (0.5)
Others	1 (0.5)
Not specified	3 (1.5)
Religion	
Islam	47 (23.7)
Christianity	147 (74.2)
Traditional	1 (0.5)
Others	1 (0.5)
Not specified	2 (1.0)

n=Total number of the respondents.

A higher proportion of those respondents from private school, when compared to those from public school, reported that tobacco ban policy is enforced in their school (73/100 versus 41/98, p-value<0.0001) (see Table 4). Lastly, a higher proportion of the males, when compared to the females supported a ban on tobacco sales to adolescents and smoking in public places (see Table 5).

Table 2. Comparison between gender of respondents and recent exposure to tobacco smoke in places where they live

Question*	Number of days	Gender*		Total
		Female	Male	
During the past 7 days, on how many days have people smoked where you live, in presence?	0	97	65	162
	1 – 2	7	6	13
	3 – 4	2	0	2
	5 – 6	0	1	1
	All 7 days	4	5	9
Total		110	77	187

p-value=0.433, df=4 (Chi-square); *Responses from 11 subjects were not computed in this statistics because they gave incomplete response to the two cross-tabulated entities.

Table 3. Comparison between gender of respondents and recent exposure to tobacco smoke in places outside where they live

Question*	Number of days	Gender*		Total
		Female	Male	
During the past 7 days, on how many days have people smoked in your presence, in places other than where you live?	0	87	67	154
	1 – 2	10	7	17
	3 – 4	3	1	4
	5 – 6	2	0	2
	All 7 days	2	5	7
Total		104	80	184

p-value=0.360, df=4 (Chi-square); *Responses from 14 respondents were not computed in this statistics because they gave incomplete response to the two cross-tabulated entities.

Table 4. Comparison between school of respondents and respondents' reports on enforcement of school smoking ban policy

Question	Response*	School		Total
		Private	Public	
Is your school's official smoking ban for school buildings enforced?	Yes, policy is enforced	73	41	114
	No, policy is not enforced	7	32	39
	School has no official ban policy	14	23	37
Total		94	96	190

p-value<0.0001, df=4 (Chi-square); *Responses from 8 respondents were not computed in this statistics because they gave incomplete response to the two cross-tabulated entities.

Table 5. Comparison between gender of respondents and attitudes toward smoking ban policy

Question*	Female (N=112)		Male (N=81)		X^2 (p-value)
	Yes	No	Yes	No	
Should tobacco sales to adolescents be banned?	59 (52.7)	48 (42.9)	45 (55.6)	32 (39.5)	0.656
Should there be a complete ban of the advertising of tobacco products?	73 (65.2)	35 (31.3)	59 (72.8)	21 (25.9)	0.361
Should smoking be banned in restaurants?	69 (61.6)	34 (30.4)	65 (80.2)	14 (17.3)	0.020
Should smoking be banned in discos/bars/pubs?	69 (61.6)	38 (33.9)	66 (81.5)	13 (16.0)	0.004
Should smoking in all enclosed public places be banned?	78 (69.6)	26 (23.2)	70 (86.4)	10 (12.3)	0.034

*Only the data of those respondents that gave complete response to the cross-tabulated entities were considered in this statistics; N=total of respondents in each category.

DISCUSSION

This study was a pilot study conducted to determine the rate of exposure of secondary school students in two selected schools in Ibokun Town, Nigeria, to secondhand tobacco smoke and also explore their attitudes towards tobacco ban policy. This study has shown that many of the surveyed students were in support of tobacco ban, while only few of them had been recently exposed to secondhand tobacco smokes.

Secondhand tobacco smokes has detrimental effects on human health (1). Unfortunately, about 1 out of every 4 secondary school students in some major Nigerian cities are exposed to these smokes (4, 5); hence making them to be at risk of developing tobacco smoke-associated diseases. In this present study, it is noteworthy that less than 15% of the respondents reported that they were exposed to secondhand tobacco within the recent seven days prior to their participation in the questionnaire. This figure is lower than that reported among their counterparts in the major Nigerian cities (4, 5). However, this study still corroborates other reports that secondhand tobacco smoke exposure is a popular experience among Nigerian school-going adolescents (4, 5).

In May 2015, the Nigerian government passed the tobacco control bill into the law, prohibiting the sales, advertisement, and consumption of tobacco and tobacco products in the Nigerian public (3). This shows that public consumption of tobacco is a criminal offence in Nigeria. In this study, authors recorded that the majority of the respondents did not approve smoking of tobacco in public places. Similar finding was also reported in a study conducted among an older population group around this study area, where 56% of the respondents in that study supported the ban of smoking in public places (7). This finding is impressive as it somehow shows a reflection of a healthy anti-smoking behavior among dwellers in the semi-urban areas in Nigeria.

Furthermore, it is noteworthy that non-enforcement of school ban policy on smoking is commonly reported among those students in the surveyed public school. Interestingly, this study was conducted 18 months after the anti-tobacco law was made in Nigeria. This concludes that the government needs to pay more attention to the enforcement of smoking ban in secondary schools.

This study has its limitations. Only the history of recent exposures to secondhand tobacco smokes were explored, this study did not explore their lifetime history of such exposures. Being a pilot study, a convenient sample size was used; this size may not be representative of the total population of secondary school students in Ibokun Town. However, authors would like to recommend if a bigger study can be conducted in this environment, covering a broader population group.

Finally, authors conclude that the rate of recent exposure to secondhand tobacco smoke among the secondary school students that participated in this study is low. Also, the enforcement of tobacco ban policy is weak in the surveyed public school. Authors therefore recommend that secondary school authorities should pay more attention to the enforcement of this policy in their schools. Lastly, the majority of the respondents were also not in support of advertisement, sales, and smoking of tobacco in public places.

ACKNOWLEDGMENTS

Authors have no competing interest to declare. This study forms part of the projects conducted in the Campaign for Head and Neck Cancer Education (CHANCE) program. The CHANCE program is an initiative of the Cephas Health Research Initiative Inc, a non-profit indigenous non-governmental organization domiciled in Nigeria.

Authors deeply appreciate the Multinational Association for Supportive Care in Cancer (MASCC) for partly funding the trip for the poster presentation of this research at the 2017 MASCC/ISOO conference which held in Washington DC, USA, in June 2017 (8). Authors also appreciate the authorities of the participating school for approving the study.

REFERENCES

[1] World Health Organization. WHO global report on trends in prevalence of tobacco smoking. Geneva: WHO, 2015.

[2] Wang L, Mamudu HM, Collins C, Wang Y. High prevalence of tobacco use and exposure to secondhand tobacco smoke among adolescents in low- and middle-income countries. Ann Transl Med 2017;5(Suppl 1):S4.

[3] Campaign for Tobacco Free Kids. Tobacco Control Laws. URL: http://www.tobaccocontrollaws.org/legislation/%20country/nigeria/laws/.

[4] Omaduvie U, Adisa A. Exposure to secondhand smoke in the home and public areas among adolescents in Abuja, Nigeria: Tobacco control implications. Tob Prev Cessation 2015 Dec 8. doi: https://doi.org/10.18332/tpc/61178.

[5] Ekanem IA. Global youth tobacco survey for Nigeria report. Calabar, Cross-River State: Department of Pathology, 2008.

[6] Wikipedia. Ibokun. URL: https://en.m.wikipedia.org/wiki/ibokun.

[7] Olowookere SA. Adepoju EG, Gbolahan OO. Awareness and attitude to the law banning smoking in public places in Osun State, Nigeria. Tob Induc Dis 2014;12(1):6.

[8] Fagbule F, Kanmodi K, Aladelusi T. Should tobacco advertisements, sales, and use be banned? – Opinions of secondary school students in Ibokun Town, State of Osun, Nigeria. Support Care Cancer 2017;25(Suppl 1):S168.

In: Childhood and Adolescence
Editor: Joav Merrick

ISBN: 978-1-53613-574-9

Chapter 11

ANAEMIA IN INFANTS: IS IT ALWAYS AN 'IRON CLAD' ISSUE? AN OBSERVATIONAL STUDY

Lutfi Jaber[1-4,*], MD and Gary Diamond[2-4], MD
[1]The Bridge to Peace Community Pediatric Center, Taibe, Israel
[2]Schneider Children's Medical Center of Israel, Petah Tikva, Israel
[3]Clalit Health Services, Tel Aviv, Israel
[4]Sackler Faculty of Medicine,
Tel Aviv University, Tel Aviv, Israel

In this chapter we examine characteristics of anaemia among infants, 9-18 months of age. Design: Comparison of trends in the characterization of anaemia in infants during the years 2002 to 2012. Setting: The comprehensive database of Clalit Health Services (CHS) for infants, divided along ethnic and religious lines. Patients: Universal screening of all infants, 9-18 months old, in the Sharon Shomron (SS) district of the CHS. Main outcome measure: Prevalence of iron deficiency anaemia (IDA). Results: Between 2002 and 2012 there was a marked decrease in IDA prevalence. Among the Jewish population, the overall IDA

* Correspondence: Professor Lutfi Jaber, MD, The Bridge to Peace Community Pediatric Center, Box 27, IL-40400 Taibe, Israel. Email: jabe@bezeqint.net.

prevalence rate dropped from 4.5% in 2002 to approximately 1.7% in 2012. The drop in prevalence was steeper in the Arab sector, where the rate plummeted from 7.0% to 2.5%. The IDA prevalence dropped by gender across ethno-religious groups from 8.8% to 3.2% for males, and 3.7% to 1.1% for females. When comparing the prevalence of anaemia by location, Pediatric Care Centers achieved greater gains against IDA than General Family Medicine Clinics. Conclusion: Mild IDA continues to exist among otherwise healthy infants, with significant declines for the 10 year period studied, with the steepest decline in the Arab community. Discrepancies remain along urban vs. rural lines. Prevention and early treatment of ID remain a priority for the child health services. IDA measures do not always reflect the true state of iron metabolism in the growing child, and added indices are proposed to better reflect the child's status.

INTRODUCTION

Iron deficiency (ID) and iron deficiency anaemia (IDA) represent a major global health problem in infants and young children (1-2). The cause of IDA among young children is multi-factorial. IDA is the most severe degree of ID. Iron depletion is the stage at which there is no storage of iron in the body. Acute aggravation of the iron balance may lead to a rapid decrease in the level of readily bio-available iron compounds. Iron deficient erythropoiesis is the stage at which the requirement of the erythroid marrow for iron is no longer fully met. At this stage, the decrease in haemogolbin (Hb) production is severe enough to lead to morphological distortion of red cells, with microcytosis and hypochromia, and the ensuing series of deleterious effects on health (3-5).

Factors associated with the increased prevalence of IDA in infants include high consumption of evaporated milk and cow's milk after six months of age, prolonged exclusive breastfeeding, and significant burden of helicobacter pylori infection (6). Other high-risk groups include children from families of low socioeconomic status (SES) (7), children of Chinese background, low-birth-weight infants, and infants who consume whole cow's milk before 12 months of age (6, 8-12). The occurrence of anaemia reportedly peaks between 6 to 24 months of age and 50% of the cases are thought to be IDA (13).

Anaemia in infants is associated with poor growth, poor development, reduced immunity, cognitive impairment and decreased stamina (14). Even more important is the evidence that the more prevalent ID, even when anaemia may not be present, may adversely affect long-term neurodevelopment and behavior, and that some of these effects may be irreversible (15). Results of randomized trials of iron supplementation in developing countries indicated that adverse effects can be prevented and/or reversed by iron supplementation early in life, or before ID becomes severe or chronic.

On the contrary McDonagh et al. (16) reported that in five of six trials no evidence was found regarding the effects of routine iron supplementation in young children on diagnosis of psychomotor, neurodevelopmental delay, or quality of life.

The prevalence of anaemia in Israel is high. When anaemia was defined as Hb level <10.5 g/dL, the prevalence was significantly higher in the Arab population (22.5%) compared with the Jewish population (10.5%) (17, 18). Over the past decade the Ministry of Health has encouraged quality, safety and upgraded service in the health system. The Clalit Health Services (CHS) adopted the recommendation to reduce the prevalence of anaemia as a health quality indicator starting in 2008 (1). In addition, they have fostered a reliable national database. This database serves the entire health system and the general public.

The purpose of this study was to utilize the comprehensive computerized database of the Clalit Health Services (CHS) to analyse the prevalence and the causative factors of IDA, as well as to characterize IDA among 9 to 18 month old Israeli infants, along SES, ethnic and geographical lines.

Our study

At present, the CHS is the largest provider of public health services in Israel (19). The CHS has computerized data. Almost all the data on medical services used by CHS members, as well as demographic characteristics, form a comprehensive database with attendant controls for assuring privacy and preventing unwarranted access (17).

Our study was conducted using the laboratory data at three arbitrary points in time for the years 2002, 2007 and 2012. The cohort comprised all infants aged 9 to 18 months for whom both the ferritin and Hb levels were evaluated. Infants suffering from chronic diseases were excluded. Data obtained included age, origin-based on residency locale and Hb and ferritin levels, number of iron preparation prescriptions dispensed to each infant by CHS pharmacies and the mother's last Hb value before giving birth.

This study design was reviewed and approved by the Human Subjects Committee of the Meir Medical Center, Kfar Saba, Israel.

Independent variables

Independent variables analyzed included age and gender. The infants' race/ethnicity included Jewish and Arab, based on locale, and designation of rural and urban residency. Socioeconomic status and weight-for-height status were not available. It was not possible to include parents' educational level and methods of feeding, since these variables were not included in the database.

Blood sampling

Blood sampling is usually performed between 9 and 14 months of age in all healthy infants. Venous blood samples were drawn from all study participants. Red blood cell indices and other parameters, were measured by the ADVIA 2120 system (20). Ferritin was analyzed using the ADVIA Centaur and ADVIA Centaur systems (21).

Definition of iron status

Serum ferritin level is the most sensitive and specific test used for the identification of ID (7).

In our study group of 9 to 18 month old infants, we defined the cut off concentration for Hb as <10.5 g/dL in children living at sea level. Haemoglobin <10.5 g/dL, ferritin <12 µg/L and mean corpuscular volume (MCV) <70 fL, were our criteria for establishing IDA, and ferritin <12 µg/L and MCV <70 fL for establishing ID. Infants whose levels of either ferritin or MCV, or both, were equal, or above these cut off points were classified as having evidence of sufficient iron intake.

Statistical analysis

Demographic parameters and relevant clinical parameters were performed using BMDP Statistical Software (22). Continuous variables were compared using analysis of variance (ANOVA) with Bonferroni's correction for multiple comparisons. We looked for correlations between various demographic variables and relevant laboratory results using Pearson's correlation. The independent variables used were ferritin, MCV and mean corpuscular hemoglobin (MCH) (absolute values). A P value of = 0.05 was considered significant.

FINDINGS

A total of 34,933 infants, aged 9-18 months, with Hb values were studied: 8,337 in 2002, 11,539 in 2007, and 15,057 in 2012. Of those, 20,779 were

Jewish and 14,154 were Arab. Grouping by gender indicated that 17,930 were males and 17,003 females. The infants' mean age at the time of the study was, 11.64 months.

In addition to the blood cell count, ferritin values were identified in 832 (10%) of the total blood tests (8,337) for 2002; 2,221 (19%) of the total blood tests (11,539) for 2007; and 2,517 (16.7%) of the total blood tests (15,057) for 2012.

Of all the 9 to 18 month old infants insured by the CHS, 27.7% were included in the study for 2002, 42.8% for 2007 and 59.4% for 2012, which indicated improved recruitment methods over the entire period studied.

Table 1. Prevalence of anaemia and iron depletion in 9 to 18 month old infants for the years 2002, 2007 and 2012

	Iron deficiency anaemia*	Iron deficiency**	Non-Iron deficiency anaemia***	Number of infants
Year 2012	N = 56 (2.22%)[a]	N = 85 (3.37%)[b]	N = 209 (8.30%)[d]	2517
Haemoglobin	9.47 ± 0.7	11.72 ± 0.67	10.02 ± 0.37	
Ferritin	6.74 ± 2.42	9.2 ± 1.5	42.14 ± 30.15	
MCV	63.18 ± 5.42	74.18 ± 2.74	74.47 ± 3.36	
Year 2007	N = 69 (3.10%)[a c]	N = 142 (6.39%)[e b]	N = 122 (5.49%)[f d]	2221
Haemoglobin	9.54 ± 0.86	11.78 ± 0.76	10.01 ± 0.44	
Ferritin	6 ± 2.47	9 ± 1.99	34 ± 20.74	
MCV	63.14 ± 4.98	73.92 ± 2.70	74.21 ± 2.92	
Year 2002	N = 54 (6.49%)[c]	N = 33 (3.96%)[e]	N = 116 (13.9%)[f]	832
Haemoglobin	9.32 ± 0.79	11.61 ± 0.63	9.89 ± 0.44	
Ferritin	7 ± 2.67	8 ± 2.33	40 ± 44.40	
MCV	63 ± 5.33	74.11 ± 3.03	74.35 ± 3.62	

MCV = mean corpuscular volume.

[a]$P = 0.06$, [b]$P < 0.001$, [c]$P < 0.001$, [d]$P < 0.001$, [e]$P = 0.01$, [f]$p < 0.001$.

*-Hb < 10.5g/dL, MCV < 70 fL, ferritin < 12 µg/L (low Hb, MCV and ferritin).

**-Hb ≥ 10.5 g/dL, MCV ≥70 fL, ferritin < 12 µg/L (normal Hb and MCV and low ferritin).

***-Hb < 10.5g/dL, ferritin > 12 µg/L.

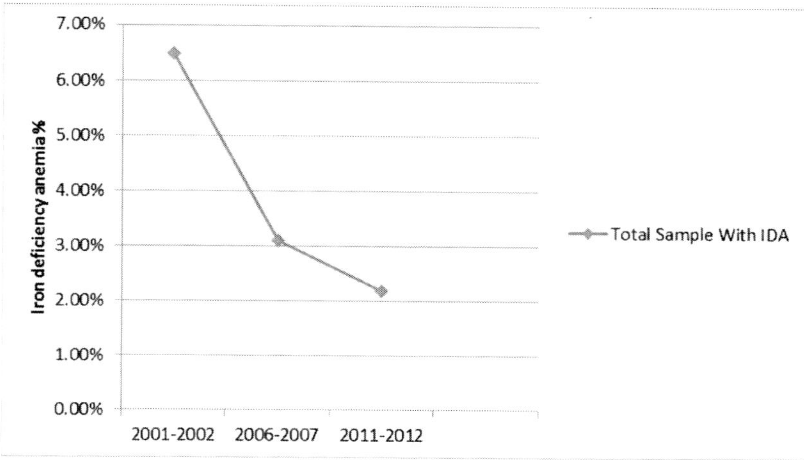

Figure 1 (a). Secular trends in iron deficiency anaemia (IDA) prevalence by year among Israeli infants aged 9 to 18 months.

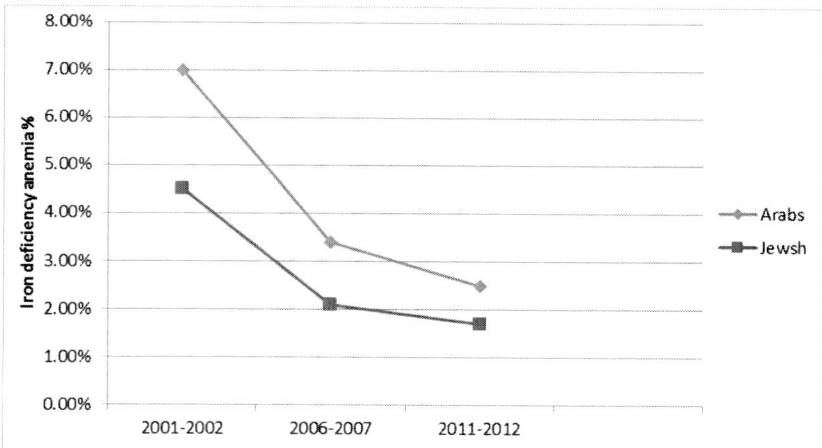

Figure 1 (b). Secular trends in iron deficiency anaemia (IDA) prevalence by sector among Israeli infants aged 9 to 18 months.

We found that for the year 2002, 6.49% of the infants had IDA, 3.96% had ID only, and 13.9% had anaemia without ID. In the year 2007. IDA, ID only, and non-IDA levels were 3.10%, 6.39%, and 5.49% respectively, whereas in 2012 the figures were 2.22%, 3.37%, and 8.3%, respectively (see Table 1).

Table 2. Changes over time in prevalence rates of iron deficiency anaemia (IDA) in Israeli infants aged 9 to 18 months. Percentage with iron deficiency in the Sharon Shomron District

Characteristic	2001-2002	2006-2007	2011-2012	Critical		Significance
Age (months)	P_1	P_2	P_3	$\lvert P_i - P_j \rvert$	p-value	
9 – 12	5.4%	3.9%	1.77%	$\lvert P_1-P_2 \rvert$	0.053	no
	(0.054)	(0.039)	(0.0177)	$\lvert P_1-P_3 \rvert$	0.047	yes
				$\lvert P_2-P_3 \rvert$	0.042	yes
12 – 15	7.2%	2.12%	3%	$\lvert P_1-P_2 \rvert$	0.053	no
	(0.072)	(0.0212)	(0.003)	$\lvert P_1-P_3 \rvert$	0.047	yes
				$\lvert P_2-P_3 \rvert$	0.027	yes
15 – 18	5.2%	6%	2.88%	$\lvert P_1-P_2 \rvert$	0.042	yes
	(0.052)	(0.006)	(0.0288)	$\lvert P_1-P_3 \rvert$	0.049	yes
				$\lvert P_2-P_3 \rvert$	0.033	yes
Ethnicity						
Arabs	7%	4.5%	2.5%	$\lvert P_1-P_2 \rvert$	0.04	yes
	(0.007)	(0.045)	(0.025)	$\lvert P_1-P_3 \rvert$	0.031	yes
				$\lvert P_2-P_3 \rvert$	0.046	yes
Jews	4.5%	2.1%	1.7%	$\lvert P_1-P_2 \rvert$	0.045	yes
	(0.045)	(0.021)	(0.017)	$\lvert P_1-P_3 \rvert$	0.043	yes
				$\lvert P_2-P_3 \rvert$	0.034	yes
Gender						
Male	8.8%	3.7%	3.2%	$\lvert P_1-P_2 \rvert$	0.061	yes
	(0.088)	(0.037)	(0.032)	$\lvert P_1-P_3 \rvert$	0.059	no
				$\lvert P_2-P_3 \rvert$	0.046	yes
Female	3.7%	2.4%	1.1%	$\lvert P_1-P_2 \rvert$	0.043	yes
	(0.037)	(0.024)	(0.011)	$\lvert P_1-P_3 \rvert$	0.038	yes
				$\lvert P_2-P_3 \rvert$	0.033	yes
Location						
Urban	7.1%	2.8%	2.4%	$\lvert P_1-P_2 \rvert$	0.054	no
	(0.071)	(0.028)	(0.024)	$\lvert P_1-P_3 \rvert$	0.053	no
				$\lvert P_2-P_3 \rvert$	0.04	yes
Rural	4.7%	3.8%	1.8%	$\lvert P_1-P_2 \rvert$	0.051	no
	(0.047)	(0.038)	(0.018)	$\lvert P_1-P_3 \rvert$	0.044	yes
				$\lvert P_2-P_3 \rvert$	0.041	yes
Pediatric Health Centers		1.2% (0.012)	1.9% (0.019)	$\lvert P_1-P_2 \rvert$	0.3173	no
General Family Medicine Clinics		3.8% (0.038)	2.3% (0.023)	$\lvert P_1-P_2 \rvert$	0.0098	yes

The characteristics of the total sample are: 6.5%, 3.1%, 2.2% for the years 2002, 2007, 2012 respectively.

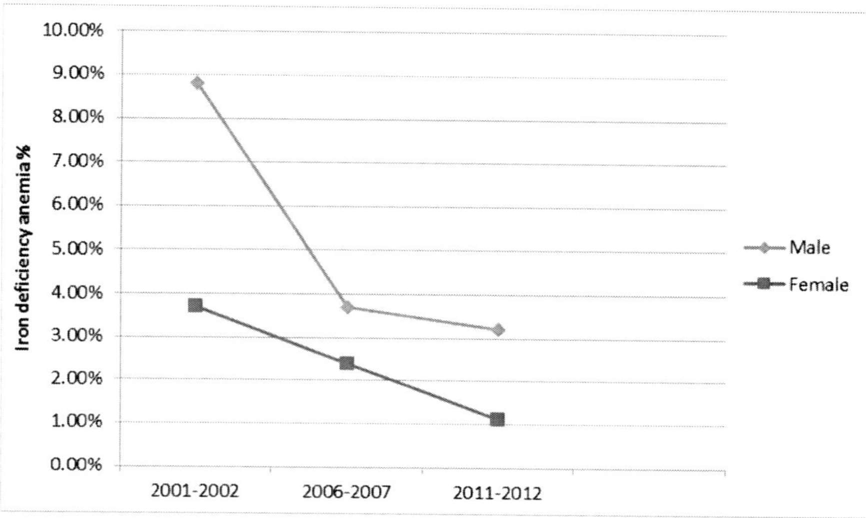

Figure 2 (a). Secular trends in iron deficiency anaemia (IDA) prevalence by gender among Israeli infants aged 9 to 18 months.

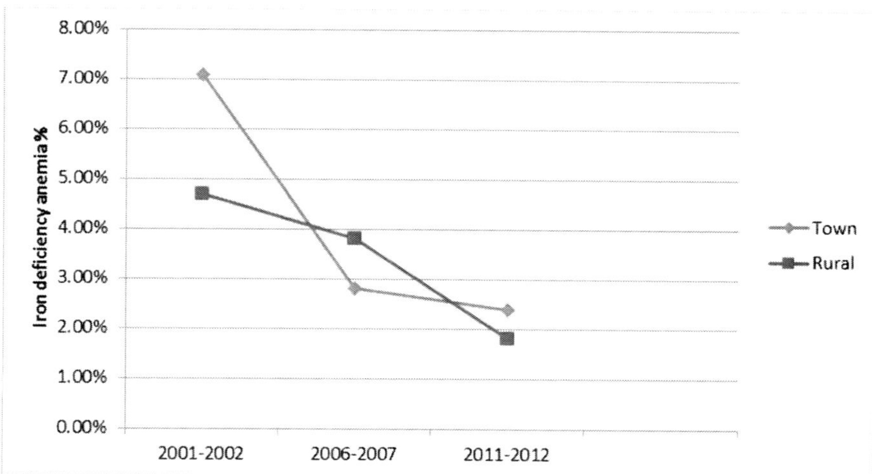

Figure 2 (b). Secular trends in iron deficiency anaemia (IDA) prevalence by location among Israeli infants aged 9 to 18 months.

The prevalence rates of IDA in the Sharon Shomron (SS) district have decreased markedly over time (see Figure 1a). The overall IDA prevalence rate in the Jewish population, since the earliest survey, dropped from 4.5%

in 2002 to 1.7% in 2012. The drop in prevalence was steepest in the Arab sector from 7.0% to 2.5% (see Table 2 and Figure 1b). This decrease occurred over two distinct periods, prior to and following the publication in 2006 of the Public Health Services directives (18).

Prevalence of IDA by gender among Israeli infants during the years 2002, 2007 and 2012 was 8.8%, 3.7%, and 3.2% for males, and 3.7%, 2.4% and 1.1% for females, respectively (see Table 2 and Figure 2a). Mean iron status indices for the year 2012 in 2,517 Israeli infants (aged 9 to 18 months) according to gender is shown in Table 3.

When comparing the prevalence of anaemia along the urban/rural divide across the whole SS district we found that for the years 2002, 2007 and 2012, the percentages were 7.1%, 2.8% and 2.4% for urban, and 4.7%, 3.8% and 1.8% for rural settings, respectively (Table 2 and Figure 2b). Lower prevalence was also found in the Pediatric Health Centers of the CHS. In the years 2007 and 2012 the percentages were 1.2% and 1.9% for the Pediatric Health Centers, and 3.8% and, 2.3% for the General Family Medicine Clinics, respectively (see Table 2).

Table 3. Mean iron status indices in 2,517 Israeli infants, aged 9 to 18-months according to gender for the years 2011 to 2012

Variable	Males (SD)	Females (SD)	*P* value	Combined (SD)
Haemoglobin	11.32 (0.97)	11.39 (0.93)	0.91	10.95 (2.30)
MCV	72.70 (5.12)	74.24 (5.26)	0.19	70.81 (14.55)
MCH	24.35 (2.14)	24.94 (2.09)	0.44	24.6 (2.14)
MCHC concentration	33.47 (1.39)	33.58 (1.28)	0.08	33.52 (1.34)
RDW	14.89 (1.45)	14.57 (1.45)	0.09	15.74 (1.46)
Ferritin	32.99 (31.18)	40.26 (38.21)	0.69	36.42 (34.86)

SD = standard deviation; MCV = mean corpuscular volume.

Discussion

This study comprehensively examined country-wide prevalence figures for IDA prevalence among Israeli infants, aged 9 to 18 months. Findings revealed that there has been an improvement in IDA prevalence among all Israeli infants, both Jewish and Arabs, during the past 12 years, with rates dropping from 6.5% to 2.2%. This incidence was found to be in the same range as the frequency reported by European countries (23-25). However, the prevalence figures skewed dramatically when the data was teased out along ethno-religious lines. The demographic and SES make-up of the Arab population is commonly that of large, low-income families, compared with the smaller and higher income families in the general Jewish sector, excluding the ultra-orthodox community. In 2007, 54.8% of the Arab population were below the poverty line (26).

Multiparty, frequent deliveries, and prolonged breastfeeding in Israel, are more common in the Arab than in the Jewish secular and modern religious population. This may partially explain the differences between both populations studied.

The IDA prevalence rates for Jews were 4.5% and 1.7%, and for Arabs 7.0% and 2.5%, respectively, for the years 2002 and 2012. These figures represent rates prior to and following publication of the Public Health directives regarding infant feeding practices, and could possibly reflect the impact of the directives on counseling for infant feeding by practitioners in the Public Health Services (18).

It should be remembered that from an historical perspective, Kaluski et al. (27) identified population group differences and reported that the prevalence has always been substantially higher in the Arab compared with the Jewish population, although the rates of decline were similar in both populations. Their cited figures had declined from approximately 70% in 1985 to approximately 30% in 1993 and to about 20% in 1996 (27).

Historically, high prevalence of IDA in Israel could be explained by ID during pregnancy, as well as:

- Infants fed a diet based on cows' milk during the first year are at greater risk for anaemia during this period
- Breast fed babies without any supplementation after the age of 6 months are similarly more prone to IDA and
- SES with its attendant nutritional characteristics (28)

The percentage of premature infants (born before 34 weeks gestational age), in the Israeli population is 8.4% of live births, and it is thought to be one of the most common causes of anaemia in infants but too statistically small to account for the rates of IDA found in our study.

The feeding of infants with iron-fortified cereals is commonplace nationwide, whereas cow's milk is not. Notably, breastfeeding in the studied community was practiced by almost 60% of Arab mothers (29). This breast fed group was also provided with preventive iron preparations. A previous study showed that the infants who were given >6 months of iron supplements starting at 4 to 6 months of age were less prone to have IDA ($P < 0.05$) (29).

In discussing comparative rates of IDA around the world, the prevalence rate of IDA in the study population in Israel is congruent with those of the Scandinavian countries and the USA. The estimated prevalence of IDA in children aged 1 to 5 years in the USA is ~1% to 2% (30-32). The incidence of IDA is also low In Norway, where only 2% to 5% of infants were found to have IDA (25).

Our values are lower than those of North American inner cities and developing countries where the prevalence of IDA in children between 6 to 24 months of age currently varies between 25 to 40% (33, 34), in China (7.8%) (35) and in Albania (47%) (36). In Estonia the values for ID and IDA were 14% and 9.4%, respectively (37). Our results are also lower when compared with those of infants aged 12 to 15 months, living in Ahwaz, a southwest area of Iran, where the prevalence of ID and IDA was 31.7% and 26.2%, respectively (38). Other recent reports studied the frequency of IDA in the Arab world: In Egypt, 64% of studied infants, aged 6 to 12 months, had IDA (39).

The prevalence of IDA in our infants in the Pediatrics Health Centers is lower than the prevalence observed in the General Family Medicine Clinics. In the Pediatrics Health Center and the General Clinics the prevalence was 1.2% versus 3.8% in the year 2007, and 1.9% versus 2.3% in the year 2012.

In our study, there was an evident correlation between the maternal Hb level detected before delivery and the frequency of IDA in their offspring. The incidence of IDA in infants born to anemic mothers is higher than in those born to nonanaemic mothers (128/659) 19% vs. (230/1414) 16%, (respectively ($P < 0.09$), which is consistent with findings by Terefe et al. (40) that maternal IDA may have an effect on the iron stores of newborns.

Children living in rural areas are more vulnerable to have more limited access to health care, and more likely to be obese than their urban counterparts. In the years 2002, 2007 and 2012, the prevalence percentages were 7.1%, 2.8% and 2.4% for urban, and 4.7%, 3.8% and 1.8% for rural settings, respectively.

Gender-based differences in iron indicators were found in Swedish (23), Icelandic (24) and Norwegian (25) studies. These studies suggested that gender-based differences are due to faster growth velocity in boys with higher iron requirements than in girls.

CONCLUSION

In summary, the low rate of IDA among our SS cohort during the last year of the survey in 2012 was unexpected, and could be attributed to several causes, such as the strict criteria that was used for establishing cut-off values for defining anaemia, as well as to the credit of the national program for the prevention of IDA (and indirectly of ID in general) in infants implemented during the later years of the survey. In addition, feeding infants with iron-fortified cereals is commonplace, and more than 60% of infants were breastfed for longer than six months, and concomitantly received recommended prophylactic iron supplementation.

Until more data becomes available, we recommend that measures should be taken to prevent overall ID, such as promoting breastfeeding at the expense of cow's milk use too early in life, using iron-fortified formula when formula is required, postponing the introduction of whole cow's milk until the end of the second year of life, and promoting the use of iron-supplemented foods, such as iron-fortified cereals. Further studies are needed for establishing valid cut-off points for diagnosing ID and IDA, and for identifying the causes of the high rate of anaemia in the absence of ID, such as haemoglobinopathies, prevalent infections during the first two years of life, and deficiencies of other nutritional factors besides that of iron.

Screening for IDA alone insufficiently reflects the true status of an infants' iron metabolism. Because of various metabolic confounding factors, iron is either present or erroneously absent, despite values for IDA, as ascertained by Hb screening alone.

Iron status being vitally important for sound physical and cognitive development, thus its evaluation should include assessment of both Hb and ferritin levels. We propose adding the ferritin measure to the national screening program for ID and anaemia in order to best reflect an infant's true potential for nutritionally-related growth and development.

REFERENCES

[1] Brotanek JM, Gosz J, Weitzman M, Flores G. Secular trends in the prevalence of iron deficiency among US toddlers, 1976-2002. Arch Pediatr Adolesc Med 2008;162:374-81.

[2] Cusick SE, Mei Z, Cogswell ME. Continuing anemia prevention strategies are needed throughout early childhood in low-income preschool children. J Pediatr 2007;150:422-8.

[3] Hercberg S, Preziosi P, Galan P. Iron deficiency in Europe. Public Health Nutr 2001;4(2B):537-45.

[4] Jain S, Kamat D. Evaluation of microcytic anemia. Clin Pediatr (Phila) 2009;48: 7-13.

[5] Baltierra D, Harper T, Jones MP, Nau KC. Hematologic disorders: Anemia. FP Essent 2015 433:11-5.

[6] Christofides A, Schauer C, Zlotkin SH. Iron deficiency anemia among children: Addressing a global public health problem within a Canadian context. Paediatr Child Health 2005;10:597-601.

[7] Camaschella C. Iron-deficiency anemia. N Engl J Med 2015; 372:1832-43.

[8] Greene-Finestone L, Feldman W, Heick H, Luke B. Prevalence and risk factors of iron depletion and iron deficiency anemia among infants in Ottawa-Carlton. Can Diet Assoc J 1991;52:20-3.

[9] Chan-Yip A, Gray-Donald K. Prevalence of iron deficiency among Chinese children aged 6 to 36 months in Montreal. Can Med Assoc J 1987;136:373- 8.

[10] Chan-Yip A, Oski FA. Consequences of starting whole cow milk at 6 months of age. J Pediatr 1987;111:813-6.

[11] Ziegler EE. Consumption of cow's milk as a cause of iron deficiency in infants and toddlers. Nutr Rev 2011;69(Suppl 1):S37-42.

[12] Oliveira MA, OsórioI MM. Cow's milk consumption and iron deficiency anemia in children. J Pediatr (Rio J) 2005;8:361-7. .

[13] Lerner NB, Sills R. Iron deficiency anemia. In: Kliegman RM, Stanton BF, St. Geme JW, Schor NF, Behrman RE, eds. Nelson textbook of pediatrics, 19th ed. Philadelphia, PA: Elsevier Saunders; 2011:1655-8.

[14] Thomas DG, Grant SL, Aubuchon-Endsley N. The role of iron in neurocognitive development. Develop Neurophsychol 2009;34:196-222.

[15] Lozoff B, Jimenez E, Smith JB. Double burden of iron deficiency in infancy and low socioeconomic status: a longitudinal analysis of cognitive test scores to age 19 years. Arch Pediatr Adolesc Med 2006,160:1108-13.

[16] McDonagh MS, Blazina I, Dana T, Cantor A, Bougatsos C. Screening and routine supplementation for Iron deficiency anemia: A systematic review. Pediatrics 2015;135:723-33. doi: 10.1542/peds.2014-3979.

[17] Meyerovitch J, Sherf M, Antebi F, Barhoum-Noufi M, Horev Z, Jaber L, et al. The incidence of anemia in an Israeli population: A population analysis for anemia in 34512 Israeli infants aged 9 to 18 months. Pediatrics 2006,118(4):e1055-60.

[18] Shalev H, Urkin J. Reduction in the prevalence of anemia in Bedouin Infants, aged 9-18 Months, in Southern Israel. Int Publ Hlth J 2014;6(1):81-4.

[19] Clalit Health Services. URL: https://en.wikipedia.org/wiki/Clalit_Health_Services).

[20] Harris N, Jou JM, Devoto G, Lotz J, Pappas J, Wranovics D, et al. Performance evaluation of the ADVIA 2120 hematology analyzer: An international multicenter clinical trial. Lab Hematol 2005,11(1):62-70.

[21] Ferritin ADVIA Centaur System. Principle of the test. UCSF Clinical Labs- Chemistry: 1-12. URL: labmed.ucsf.edu/labmanual/db/resource/Centaur_ Ferritin.pdf.

[22] Dixon WJ, ed. BMDP Statistical Software. Los Angeles, CA: University of California Press, 1993.

[23] Domello FM, Hernell O. Iron-deficiency anaemia during the first two years of life. Scand J Nutr 2002;46:20-30.

[24] Thorsdottir I, Gunnarsson BS, Atladottir H, Michaelsen KF, Palsson G. Iron status at 12 months of age – effects of body size, growth and diet in population with high birth weight. Eur J Clin Nutrition 2003;57:505-13.

[25] Hay G, Sandstad B, Whitelaw A, Borch-Iohnsen B. Iron status in a group of Norwegian children aged 6–24 months. Acta Paediatr 2004,93(5):592-8.

[26] Halabi R. Poverty in an Israeli Arab population. Zichron: The Center for Political Economics; 2007:167–171. URL: http:// www.macro.org.il/lib/File/Zichron% 20book%202008/Halabi.pdf.

[27] Kaluski DN, Leventhal A, Averbuch Y, Rishpon S, Cohen-Dar M, Habib S, et al. Five decades of trends in anemia in Israeli infants: implications for food fortification policy. Eur J Clin Nutr 2001;55(2):82-7.

[28] Oski FA. Iron deficiency in infancy and childhood. N Engl J Med 1993;329:190-3.

[29] Jaber L. Preventive intervention for iron deficiency anaemia in a high risk population. Int J Risk Saf Med 2014;26:155-62.

[30] Siu AL, on behalf of the US Preventive Services Task Force. Screening for iron deficiency anemia in young children: USPSTF Recommendation Statement. Pediatrics 2015;136;746-52. doi: 10.1542/peds.2015-2567.

[31] Baker RD, Greer FR, Committee on Nutrition American Academy of Pediatrics. Diagnosis and prevention of iron deficiency and iron-deficiency anemia in infants and young children (0-3 years of age). Pediatrics 2010;126:1040-50. doi: 10.1542/peds.2010-2576.

[32] Cusick SE, Mei Z, Freedman DS, Looker AC, Ogden CL, Gunter E, et al. Unexplained decline in the prevalence of anemia among US children and women between 1988-1994 and 1999-2002. Am J Clin Nutr 2008;88(6):1611-7.

[33] Booth IW, Aukett MA. Iron deficiency anaemia in infancy and early childhood. Arch Dis Child 1997,76:549-54.

[34] Gregory JR, Collins DL, Davies PSW, Hughes JM, Clarke PC. National Diet and Nutrition survey: Children aged 1½ to 4½ years. Volume 1: Report of the Diet and Nutrition Survey. London: HMSO, 1995.

[35] Zhu YP, Liao QK. Collaborative Study Group for the Epidemiological Survey of Iron Deficiency in Children in China. Prevalence of iron deficiency in children aged 7 months to 7 years in China. Hematol J 2005,5:579-83.

[36] Buonomo E, Cenko F, Altan AM, Godo A, Marazzi, Palombi L. Iron deficiency anemia and feeding practices in Albanian children. Ann Ig 2005,17(1):27-33.

[37] Vendt N, Grünberg H, Leedo S, Tillmann V, Talvik T. Prevalence and causes of iron deficiency anemias in infants aged 9 to 12 months in Estonia. Medicina (Kaunas) 2007,43:947-52.

[38] Monajemzadeh SM, Zarkesh MR. Iron deficiency anemia in infants aged 12-15 months in Ahwaz, Iran. Indian J Pathol Microbiol 2009,52:182-4.

[39] Al Ghwass MM, Halawa EF, Sabry SM, Ahmed D. Iron deficiency anemia in an Egyptian pediatric population: A cross-sectional study. Ann Afr Med 2015;14:25-31.

[40] Terefe B, Birhanu A, Nigussie P, Tsegaye A. Effect of maternal iron deficiency anemia on the iron store of newborns in Ethiopia. Anemia 2015;2015:808204. doi: 10.1155/2015/808204.

In: Childhood and Adolescence
Editor: Joav Merrick

ISBN: 978-1-53613-574-9

Chapter 12

Child abuse and alcohol misuse in a victim: The role of ethnic and societal factors

Sergei V Jargin*[*], *MD
Peoples' Friendship University of Russia, Moscow, Russia

The case report describes a co-occurrence of child abuse, autistic symptoms, and excessive alcohol consumption in the victim's adolescence and early adulthood. The conclusion is that environmental factors such as physical and psychological abuse may contribute to the appearance of autistic traits. Abnormal behaviors partly compatible with the autism spectrum disorder (ASD) may be adaptive. Alcohol is consumed by some autistic adolescents to maintain friendships and gain access to relationships. Besides, loitering with groups of juvenile alcohol consumers is a way of escape from domestic violence. The role of ethnicity-related and other societal factors is discussed.

---

[*] Correspondence: Sergei V Jargin, MD, Peoples' Friendship University of Russia, Clementovski per 6-82, 115184 Moscow, Russia. Email: sjargin@mail.ru.

INTRODUCTION

There is considerable evidence demonstrating associations between childhood trauma, including physical, sexual and emotional abuse, with negative mental, physical health and social outcomes, deficient communicative skills, substance abuse and in particular misuse of alcohol in a victim's later life (1-4). The prevalence of the substance use among individuals with autism was reported to be relatively low (5); although underestimation is not excluded (6). People with high-functioning autism may drink alcohol to cope with anxiety, to maintain friendships and gain access to new relationships (6, 7). Furthermore, the youth with autism spectrum disorder (ASD) were found to be at a higher risk of victimization and bullying (8-12). Given the association of autistic traits in adults with the abuse in their childhood, studies identifying causal mechanisms can improve preventive efforts (13). Here is presented a case illustrating a combination of the above-named symptoms and factors as a continuation of the case report (4).

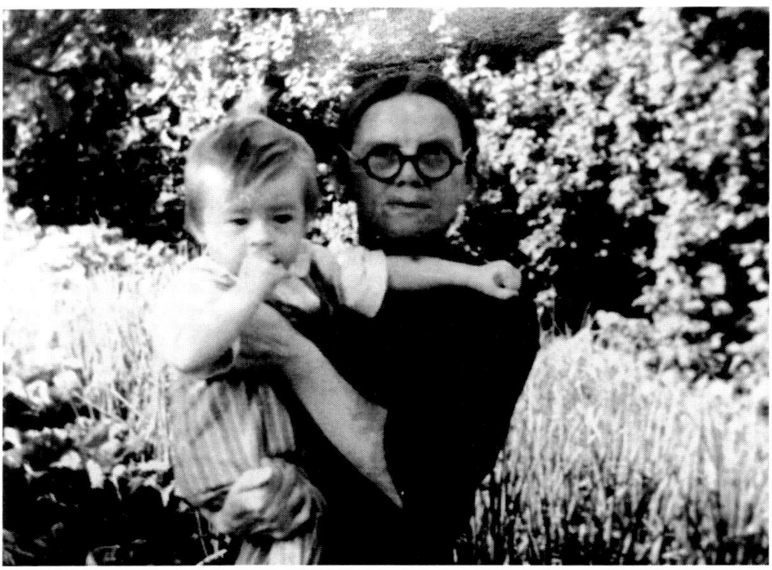

Figure 1. Sergei age about one year and his nanny Alexandra age 53 years.

CASE REPORT

When Sergei (S) was three years old, his parents were divorced, while he was sent with a nanny to a suburb village. They spent there also two subsequent summers, having almost no contact with other children. The boy sat on a sofa or bench on end, which did not contribute to his physical development and communicative skills. Once the father came unexpectedly and smelled alcohol: the nanny gave to S sweet fortified wine as "cough mixture" probably to calm him down and not to be disturbed at night. No action was taken by the father (see Figure 1).

At the age of around six years, S was noticed to have autistic traits: communication deficits, failure to develop peer relationships and motor clumsiness. Some features compatible with the ADHD (attention deficit hyperactivity disorder) were observed as well: inattention, impulsivity and hyperactivity, the latter being more pronounced in a familiar environment. Appearance of the autistic symptoms coincided with the time when the socially unskilled child was exposed to bullying; the symptoms further aggravated in parallel with the physical abuse at home. Besides, it should be mentioned that S has a relative macrocephaly (head circumference at an adult age approximately 60.5 cm), similarly to his mother and father, who both were professors. An increased prevalence of macrocephaly has been described in children with ASD (14, 15). Some researchers reported a higher level of functioning in children with ASD and macrocephaly in comparison to those with average head circumference (16). Moderately expressed marfanoid features (long limbs, arachnodactyly, hypermobility of some joints, hiatal hernia in a later life) were noticed in S and in some maternal relatives. An association of macrocephaly, Marfan-like ligamentous laxity and Asperger's syndrome has been reported (17).

When S was seven years old, his mother married a relative, who was 15 years older than S. The stepfather turned out to be a child abuser. An ethnic factor could have played a role: the stepfather was of Jewish descent, while S used to stress his Russian ethnicity. His father and maternal grandfather were both ethnic Russians, while the maternal grandmother was of Jewish descent at least in part. The abuse was administered by slapping in the face and head as well as beating with a belt, often under the pretext of punishment, but sometimes without any pretext whatever. Episodes of violence went along with intimidation by gestures and mimic (2, 4). By the age 8-9 years, the above-mentioned autistic traits had become prominent, were noticed at school and obviously contributed to the bullying.

Admittedly, there was another factor that might have contributed to the abnormal behavior, although a cause-effect relationship is by no means proven. The onset of the behavioral abnormalities coincided with the UHF (ultrahigh frequency) therapy for allergic rhinitis and tonsillitis repeatedly at the age 4-6.5 years. Slight but persistent dysphagia was noticed at the same time. The therapy with ultrahigh frequency electromagnetic fields has been officially recommended in the former Soviet Union and broadly used in otorhinolaryngolical practice since the early 1960s (18, 19). Last time, the extremely high frequency (EHF) waves have also been used for respiratory and allergic conditions in children, while absence of contraindications has been pointed out (20). At the same time, reports on non-thermal effects of electromagnetic waves from anthropogenic sources, in particular, functional derangements of the nervous system, have appeared (21, 22); the reported results, however, were not always reproducible (23). Note that doses of thermal intensity used in the UHF therapy are higher than those from anthropogenic environmental sources, causing no measurable temperature increase of living tissues. Considering anatomical proximity of tonsils, nasal cavity and neural structures especially in children, there have been concerns about such use of electromagnetic waves, the more so as excessive exposures and imprecise focusing may occur in the therapeutic routine. Subjective factors of different kind cannot be excluded: S was regularly brought to the polyclinics by his Jewish grandmother, so that medical personnel knew them both very well. Subsequently, at the age of 6-7 years, S underwent tonsillectomy and adenoidectomy with questionable indications and insufficient local anesthesia. Later it has become evident that he had allergic rhinitis. The grandmother herself had undergone hysterectomy and

Halsted mastectomy with questionable indications and complications - enlarging postoperative hernia, chronic pain and edema. Ethnicity-related factors might have been active also in this connection (3).

Having a Jewish stepfather, who even worked for some period at his school, S was often treated by the social environment as a member of the ethnic minority. It apparently contributed to the bullying, sometimes visibly inspired by adults including some teachers and other children's relatives. The bullying generally happened at schools, where children did not feel safe to report bullies (24). The author does not intend to say that Jewish children were generally bullied at Soviet schools. Many of them were not, as they had been prepared by their families and did not deny their difference. On the contrary, S behaved ambitiously, involuntarily provoking his environment. S himself participated in bullying other children, his role thus being classified as bully-victim, reportedly more at risk of substance use than pure bullies or victims (25). Other factors potentially contributing to the alcohol consumption has been discussed previously (4).

Apart from occasional participation in parties at home and drinking up to a bottle of beer with a schoolmate, S did not consume alcohol till the age of 13 years. That summer he drank a 0.75 l bottle of fortified wine with an older boy. During the subsequent year, his alcohol consumption increased up to 250 ml of vodka with beer or a 0.75 l bottle of fortified wine at one session. An opportunity to stay away from domestic violence was provided by a drinking company of schoolmates including older boys inspiring alcohol purchase and consumption. During the following years, he was several times detained by the police (militia) and spent at least two nights at a sobering-up station. At the age of 13.5 years, S ran away from the violence first to his grandmother and then lived about two years in a small apartment together with the new family of his father. Thereafter he was manipulated to return to the mother's flat. After the admission to a university, a separate room was rented for S. Next year he was dismissed from the university and served two years with the army; his education was interrupted for four years. The immediate cause of the dismissal was as follows. Having worked two months with a students' construction brigade (stroyotriad), after a provocation from the social environment and excessive alcohol intake, S went with a companion to the Black Sea, where he was robbed and remained without money for a return ticket. Despite repeated telegrams and telephone calls, he received money with a delay, which resulted in about two weeks' tardiness at the university. At the age of about 22.5 years, S underwent an implantation of the disulphiram preparation Esperal®, which was followed by a period of abstinence of about eight months. After that he resumed alcohol consumption: 2-3 binges monthly with dosages as described above or higher. S discontinued the alcohol misuse at the age of about 35 years, when it has become incompatible with his professional duties. Later he did not resume the excessive alcohol consumption in spite of provocations from the social environment. With time, subconscious motives of the alcohol intake have become clear: alcohol helped him to overcome communication barriers. It was, however, associated with risks: not possessing sufficient social skills, his rhetoric and actions under the impact of alcohol were sometimes precarious (26). This illustrates the mechanism contributing to the alcohol consumption not only in autistic individuals: becoming "insider" through drinking with peers. This mechanism has been exploited: in workers', students' and intelligentsia companies, ringleaders were observed, who manipulated others towards alcohol intake, while non-drinkers were sometimes stigmatized (27).

To finish the case report on an optimistic note, it should be mentioned that S made conscious efforts to forgive the abusers. The mother and her partner cooperated with the author of this report in elucidation of the motives, of psychological, ethnic and social aspects of child abuse. In particular, according to the mother's memory, behavioral and communication abnormalities during Sergei's preschool time coincided with bullying on the playgrounds near their apartment house, which was apparently in some cases inspired by adults and tolerated by his nanny.

DISCUSSION

The ASD cases are often marked by symptoms consistent with ADHD (28-30). In the case presented here, some ADHD symptoms were observed especially during the early childhood: inattention, impulsivity and hyperactivity, the latter being more prominent in a familiar environment. Appearance and worsening of the autistic symptoms coincided with the time when the socially unskilled child was exposed to the bullying and domestic violence. In the author's opinion, physical abuse is an undervalued cause of autism. Some children with autistic symptoms are probably abused ADHD or initially healthy children, possibly having unusual traits predisposing to the bullying. In the atmosphere of bullying and domestic violence, ADHD manifestations such as impulsivity and hyperactivity may be regularly punished. Abnormal behavior seems to be a kind of adaptation in some cases, a consciously or subconsciously implemented strategy to avoid the maltreatment. Such behavior might be compatible with the ASD: a failure to respond to social interactions, poorly integrated communication, abnormalities of eye contact, deficits of developing and maintaining relationships (DSM-5). Deranged relationship with parents as a known ASD manifestation can be a consequence of child abuse. Avoidance of eye contacts may result from intimidation. Interestingly, the avoidance of eye contacts was not noticed in S till the age of about 13 years, when a teacher told Sergei's mother that the boy had an "insolent gaze"; and the mother instructed him not to look into peoples' eyes. An association of both ASD and ADHD with deranged relationships with parents, maternal stress and child abuse has been reported (13, 31, 32). Other features compatible with the ASD may be secondary to a deficit in relationships with peers and relatives or result from sublimation as a defense mechanism against anxiety and psychological trauma (28), e.g., fixated interests such as the study of special subjects beyond the school program.

According to the hypothesis discussed here, some ASD cases may be caused by intrinsic factors while others are induced or reinforced by environmental factors such as the physical abuse and bullying. ADHD, ASD and social anxiety disorder have partly overlapping symptoms (29, 30, 33, 34). A differentiation may depend on external factors: in an environment permitting impulsivity and hyperactivity, the child would preserve ADHD features or develop in a typical way. In conditions of bullying and domestic violence, regularly punishing impulsivity and hyperactivity, the child might be "educated" towards abnormal behaviors aimed at avoidance of the trauma. It can also be speculated that children with macrocephaly consciously or subconsciously protect their heads. On the other hand, macrocephaly, "giftedness" (35), marfanoid or other unusual features might predispose to the bullying. The cause-effect relationship may be bidirectional: autistic symptoms can enhance the risk of domestic violence and bullying, while the violence would induce and reinforce abnormal behaviors. In conclusion, the child abuse and bullying may be causative factors of atypical behaviors more or less compatible with the ASD.

REFERENCES

[1] Springer KW, Sheridan J, Kuo D, Carnes M. The long-term health outcomes of childhood abuse. An overview and a call to action. J Gen Intern Med 2003;18: 864-70.

[2] Jargin SV. Child abuse and alcohol misuse in a victim. Alcoh Alcohol 2011;46:734-6.

[3] Jargin SV. Elder abuse and neglect versus parricide. Int J High Risk Behav Addict 20132(3):136-8.

[4] Jargin SV. Child abuse and alcohol misuse in a victim: The role of ethnic and societal factors. Int J Child Adolesc health 2013;6(3):351-5.

[5] Ramos M, Boada L, Moreno C, Llorente C, Romo J, Parellada M. Attitude and risk of substance use in adolescents diagnosed with Asperger syndrome. Drug Alcohol Depend 2013;133:535-40.

[6] Lalanne L, Weiner L, Trojak B, Berna F, Bertschy G. Substance-use disorder in high-functioning autism: clinical and neurocognitive insights from two case reports. BMC Psychiatry 2015;15:149.

[7] Rengit AC, Mc Kowen JW, O'Brien J, Howe YJ, McDougle CJ. Brief report: Autism spectrum disorder and substance use disorder: A review and case study. J Autism Dev Disord 2016;46:2514-9.

[8] Zablotsky B, Bradshaw CP, Anderson CM, Law P. Risk factors for bullying among children with autism spectrum disorders. Autism 2014;18:419-27.

[9] Hebron J, Oldfield J, Humphrey N. Cumulative risk effects in the bullying of children and young people with autism spectrum conditions. Autism 2017;21:291-300.

[10] Maïano C, Normand CL, Salvas MC, Moullec G, Aimé A. Prevalence of school bullying among youth with autism spectrum disorders: A systematic review and meta-analysis. Autism Res 2016;9:601-15.

[11] Sterzing PR, Shattuck PT, Narendorf SC, Wagner M, Cooper BP. Bullying involvement and autism spectrum disorders: prevalence and correlates of bullying involvement among adolescents with an autism spectrum disorder. Arch Pediatr Adolesc Med 2012;166:1058-64.

[12] Zeedyk SM, Rodriguez G, Tipton LA, Baker BL, Blacher J. Bullying of youth with autism spectrum disorder, intellectual disability, or typical development: Victim and parent perspectives. Res Autism Spectr Disord 2014;8:1173-83.

[13] Roberts AL, Koenen KC, Lyall K, Robinson EB, Weisskopf MG. Association of autistic traits in adulthood with childhood abuse, interpersonal victimization, and posttraumatic stress. Child Abuse Negl 2015;45:135-42.

[14] Aylward EH, Minshew NJ, Field K, Sparks BF, Singh N. Effects of age on brain volume and head circumference in autism. Neurology 2002;59:75-183.

[15] Sacco R, Gabriele S, Persico AM. Head circumference and brain size in autism spectrum disorder: A systematic review and meta-analysis. Psychiatry Res 2015;234:239-51.

[16] Zachor DA, Ben-Itzchak E. Specific medical conditions are associated with unique behavioral profiles in autism spectrum disorders. Front Neurosci 2016;10:410.

[17] Tantam D, Evered C, Hersov L. Asperger's syndrome and ligamentous laxity. J Am Acad Child Adolesc Psychiatry 1990;29:892-6.

[18] Nikolaevskaia VP. The use of microwave therapy in patients with chronic tonsillitis. Vestn Otorinolaringol 1966;(6):31-4.

[19] Nikolaevskaia VP. Microwave therapy of ear, nose and throat diseases. Methodical letter. Health Ministry of RSFSR, Moscow 1966. [Russian]

[20] Povazhnaia EL, Mambetalieva AS. Extremely high frequency therapy for the prevention of acute respiratory diseases in children with chronic ENT and allergic diseases. Vopr Kurortol Fizioter Lech Fiz Kult 2010;(5):170-21.

[21] Shandala MG. Experience in a hygienic assessment of problems related to physical environmental factors. Gig Sanit 1999;(4):3-9.

[22] Shandala MG. Physical environmental factors in the ecology of the brain. Gig Sanit 2015;(3):10-14.

[23] McRee DI. Review of Soviet/Eastern European research on health aspects of microwave radiation. Bull NY Acad Med 1979;55:11330-51.

[24] LePage P, Courey S. Teaching children with high-level autism. London: Routledge, 2014.

[25] Radliff KM, Wheaton JE, Robinson K, Morris J. Illuminating the relationship between bullying and substance use among middle and high school youth. Addict Behav 2012;37:569-72.

[26] Jargin SV. Letter from Russia: alcoholism and dissent-report of a whistleblower. Alcohol Alcohol 2011;46:498-9.

[27] Jargin SV. On the causes of alcoholism in the former Soviet Union. Alcohol Alcohol 2010;45:104-5.

[28] Metzger JA. Adaptive defense mechanisms: function and transcendence. J Clin Psychol 2014;70:478-88.

[29] Hartley SL and Sikora DM. Which DSM-IV-TR criteria best differentiate high-functioning autism spectrum disorder from ADHD and anxiety disorders in older children? Autism 2009;13:485-509.

[30] Mayes SD. Checklist for autism spectrum disorder. Chicago, IL: Stoelting, 2012.

[31] Weber-Börgmann I, Burdach S, Barchfeld P, Wurmser H. Associations with ADHD and parental distress with disinterest in play in early childhood. Z Kinder Jugendpsychiatr Psychother 2014;42:147-55.

[32] Duan G, Chen J, Zhang W, Yu B, Jin Y, Wang Y, Yao M. Physical maltreatment of children with autism in Henan province in China: A cross-sectional study. Child Abuse Negl 2015;48:140-7.

[33] Murray MJ. Attention-deficit/Hyperactivity Disorder in the context of Autism spectrum disorders. Curr Psychiatr Rep 2010;12:382-8.

[34] Kleberg JL, Högström J, Nord M, Bölte S, Serlachius E, Falck-Ytter T. Autistic traits and symptoms of social anxiety are differentially related to attention to others' eyes in social anxiety disorder. J Autism Dev Disord 2016 Dec 20. doi: 10.1007/s10803-016-2978-z.

[35] Miller A. The drama of the gifted child. New York: Basic Books, 2008.

In: Childhood and Adolescence
Editor: Joav Merrick

ISBN: 978-1-53613-574-9

Chapter 13

INCIDENTAL ORAL HAIRY LEUCOPLAKIA (OHL) IN A HEALTHY ASYMPTOMATIC INDIVIDUAL

Lyubov Matytsina-Quinlan[1,*], MD, PhD, DM, DFSRH, Mrinalini Mahto[1], MD, Donald E Greydanus[2], MD, DrHC (Athens) and Laura Gwatkin[1,3], MD

[1]East Cheshire Centre for Sexual Health, East Cheshire NHS Trust, Macclesfield District General Hospital, Macclesfield, Cheshire, United Kingdom

[2]Department of Pediatric and Adolescent Medicine, Western Michigan University Homer Stryker MD School of Medicine, Kalamazoo, Michigan, US

[3]Aneurin Bevan Health Board, Nevill Hall Hospital, Abergavenny, Wales, United Kingdom

[*] Correspondence: Lyubov Matytsina-Quinlan, MD, PhD, DM, DFSRH, East Cheshire Centre for Sexual Health, East Cheshire NHS Trust, Macclesfield District General Hospital, Macclesfield, Cheshire, SK103BL, United Kingdom. Email: lyubov.matytsina@yahoo.com.

This report highlights oral hairy leukoplakia (OHL) in a healthy asymptomatic individual. A heterosexual man in his 20s was referred by his doctor for human immunodeficiency virus (HIV) testing with bilateral non-painful persistent whitish lesions on his tongue. Examination revealed bilateral whitish non-removable lesions along the lateral tongue borders consistent with OHL. Routine screening tests for sexually transmitted infections (STIs) including human immunodeficiency virus (HIV) were all negative along with complete blood count (CBC), urea, electrolytes and liver function tests (LFTs). Serology for the Epstein-Barr virus (EBV) was consistent with previous EBV infection. Histology confirmed OHL. OHL can occur in asymptomatic healthy HIV-negative individuals but it is important to exclude specific causes of immunosuppression.

Introduction

We present a rare cause of oral hairy leukoplakia (OHL) in a young asymptomatic heterosexual patient at low risk of sexually transmitted infections (STIs) and HIV. OHL is associated with Epstein-Barr virus (EBV) infection and is mostly found in immune-compromised patients such as human immunodeficiency virus (HIV) or in patients with transplants and haematological malignancies. This case report highlights that OHL can also occur in healthy asymptomatic individuals. However, before concluding this, causes of immunosuppression need to be excluded by routine blood tests, sexually transmitted infection (STI) screening and or biopsy.

Case report

A 26-year old male was referred by his general practitioner to the Genitourinary Medicine (GUM) Department with persistent whitish lesions on the borders of his tongue for exclusion of HIV infection. He was an otherwise asymptomatic heterosexual male with his last sexual intercourse two years ago. He gave a history of whitish lesions on his tongue first being noticed by his dentist nine months earlier. He did not give any history of weight loss or any influenza-like symptoms and had no genitourinary symptoms.

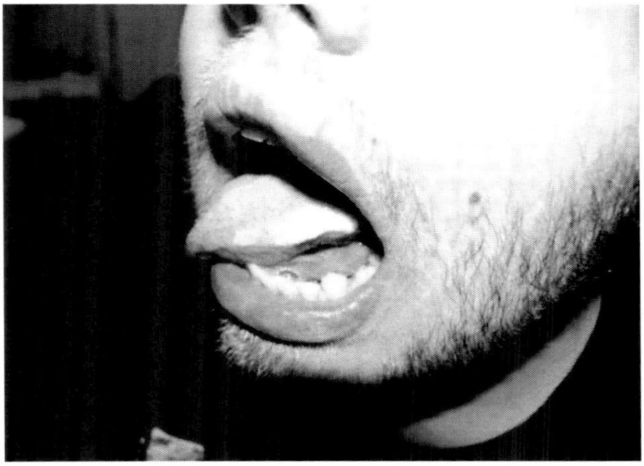

Figure 1. Whitish lesions on 26-year old male.

Past medical and family history were unremarkable and he was not on any type of prescribed or over-the-counter medication. He denied smoking, chewing tobacco, taking alcohol, injecting drugs or ever having taking steroids. He gave no history of drug allergies. He denied having sex with men and also denied having sex abroad or commercial sex. He last had protected vaginal sex with his ex-girlfriend two years ago and had no history of STIs. He gave no history of any lesions elsewhere and had no oral or genitourinary symptoms. He did not have any tattoos or any body piercings.

Examination of the oral cavity revealed bilateral whitish non-removal plaques along the lateral tongue borders consistent with OHL (see Figure 1). Characteristic raised lesions were adherent and were not removed by scraping. There was no associated erythema or edema of the surrounding tissue. On the dorsal part of the tongue were typical "hairy" appearance of whitish lesions while on the ventral part of the tongue, the lesions were slightly lacking the characteristic hairy appearance of OHL. The result of examination and clinical presentation were highly suggestive of hairy leukoplakia. There was no other finding on oral examination. General, systemic and genital examinations were all normal.

Routine STI screening tests were negative. These tests included urine nucleic acid amplification test (NAAT) for Neisseria gonorrhoeae and Chlamydia trachomatis as well as blood tests for syphilis and HIV. Serology for the Epstein-Barr (EBV) virus was consistent with EBV infection in the past (more than eight months). Routine blood tests in the form of complete blood count (CBC), electrolytes and liver function tests were all normal.

Biopsy of the lesions with histological investigation confirmed OHL. The sections showed marked squamous hyperplasia with prominent hyperparakeratosis and perinuclear clearing. A dense surface coat of bacteria is evident superficially, but candida was not found. There was no evidence of malignancy or atypia. The histological features were suggestive of hairy leukoplakia. The differential diagnoses included oral candidiasis, lichen planus, tobacco-associated leukoplakia, morsicatio mucosae oris, squamous cell carcinoma and human papillomavirus (HPV) induced neoplasia.

The patient was treated with valacyclovir 1,000 milligrams three times a day for two weeks. He did not develop any side effects to the treatment; however, his lesions still persisted at an examination one month later. He was advised to return, but was lost to follow-up.

DISCUSSION

Oral hairy leucoplakia (OHL) is a disease of the mucosa firstly described in 1984 (1). It is caused by EBV infection, is seen in immune compromised patients and is considered a marker of immunosuppression. OHL associated with EBV mostly occurs in HIV patients (2). OHL is a rare condition in healthy individuals and can also be present in healthy, asymptomatic HIV negative individuals with past EBV infection.

EBV is a herpes virus and has been associated with a number of diseases, mainly in immune-compromised patients. It is usually symptomless unless there is super infection of Candida (3). Culture investigation can be performed when clinically indicated and especially in HIV-positive individuals as well as immuno-compromised patients. OHL is found in immune-suppressed and immuno-compromised patients such as HIV/AIDS, haematological malignancies, transplant cases and those on steroids (3-6).

It has also has been described in association with Behcet's syndrome (7) and ulcerative colitis (1). OHL lesions can be confused with candidiasis; however, in candidiasis lesions can be easily scraped off (8). Other differential diagnoses included lichen planus, tobacco-associated leucoplakia, squamous cell carcinoma and human papillomavirus (HPV) – induced neoplasia (1). Biopsy will help to establish the diagnosis. OHL in iatrogenically immune-suppressed patients can respond to withdrawal of immune-suppressive medications.

It is important that STIs screening (including HIV testing), routine blood tests and biopsy of the lesion(s) be performed to exclude other causes. Also, investigation for EBV is important as EBV leads to recurring infection of the intraoral epithelium (9). Generally, treatment for OHL is not required; however, it may be resolved with anti-herpes medication (i.e., acyclovir or valacyclovir) in HIV-negative patients. It is important to treat any underlying causes, as for example antiretroviral agents in HIV patients (2, 10).

In our case, the patient was treated with valcyclovir (1,000 mgs TDS for two weeks) and followed up in one month. His lesions persisted and he did not attend his further follow-up appointment. OHL is a very rare condition in HIV negative healthy individuals.

There are not many cases of bilateral OHL reported in non-immunosuppressed HIV negative males. Those cases reported in HIV negatives in literature were mainly in those who had been on steroids.

We did not find a similar published case in the literature, but found a commentary on the British Medical Journal (BMJ) website citing an article by Scully and Porter on this topic (10). A review of the literature notes that

OHL does not confirm that the patient has HIV/AIDs (1-11). Our report highlights that OHL can occur in HIV negative, healthy and asymptomatic individuals. However, before one concludes this, it is important to exclude causes of immunosuppression such as HIV or long term steroid use. We thus conclude that OHL can represent an isolated and innocuous EBV infection. Nevertheless, it is important to exclude all known causes associate with OHL.

CONCLUSION

OHL is associated with EBV and is found in immuno-compromised patients such as HIV and/or HIV/AIDS, haematological malignancies, transplant cases and those on steroids; it also has been described in association with Behcet's syndrome, as well as ulcerative colitis. OHL rarely can occur in immune-competent, HIV-negative healthy individuals. It is important to exclude all known causes associated with OHL including HIV by STI screening, routine blood tests and biopsy of the lesion.

ACKNOWLEDGMENTS

Our patient was not involved in a clinical trial and no competing interest occurred. Patient consent was obtained.

REFERENCES

[1] Lynch DP. Hairy leukoplakia: Background, pathophysiology, epidemiology. URL: https://emedicine.medscape.com/article/279269-overview.

[2] Pattman R, Snow M, Handy P, Sankar KN, Elawad B, eds. Oxford handbook of genitourinary medicine, HIV, and sexual health. Oxford: Oxford University Press, 2005.

[3] McMillan IR, Young H, Ogilvie MM, Scott G, eds. Clinical practice in sexually transmitted infections. London: Saunders, 2002.

[4] Graboyes EM, Allen CT, Chernock RD, Diaz JA. Oral hairy leukoplakia in an HIV-negative patient. Ear Nose Throat J 2013:92(6):E12.

[5] Blomgren J, Bäck H. Oral hairy leukoplakia in a patient with multiple myeloma. Oral Surg Oral Med Oral Pathol Oral Radiol Endod 1996;82(4):408-10.

[6] Piperi E, Omlie J, Koutlas IG, Pambuccian S. Oral hairy leukoplakia in a HIV-negative patients: Report of 10 cases. Int J Surg Pathol 2010;18(3):177-83.

[7] Schiodt M, Norgaard T, Greenspan JS. Oral hairy leukoplakia in a HIV-negative woman with Behcet's syndrome. Oral Surg Oral Med Oral Pathol Oral Radiol Endod 1995;79(1):53-6.

[8] Morse SA, Ballard RC, Holmes KK, Moreland AA, eds. Atlas of sexually transmitted diseases and AIDS, 4th ed. London: Saunders Elsevier, 2010.

[9] Itin PH. Oral hairy leukoplakia-10 years on. Dermatology 1993;187(3):159-63.

[10] Scully C, Porter S. ABC of oral health. Swelling and red, white, and pigmented lesions BMJ 2000;321(7255):225-8.

[11] Greenspan D, Greenspan JS, Hearst NG, Pan LZ, Conant MA, Abrams DI, et al. Relation of oral hairy leucoplakia to infection with the human immunodeficiency virus and the risk of developing AIDS. J Infect Dis 1987;155(3):475-81.

Section two: Acknowledgments

In: Childhood and Adolescence
Editor: Joav Merrick

ISBN: 978-1-53613-574-9

Chapter 14

About the Author

Joav Merrick, MD, MMedSci, DMSc, born and educated in Denmark is professor of pediatrics, child health and human development, Division of Pediatrics, Hadassah Hebrew University Medical Center, Mt Scopus Campus, Jerusalem, Israel and Kentucky Children's Hospital, University of Kentucky, Lexington, Kentucky United States and professor of public health at the Center for Healthy Development, School of Public Health, Georgia State University, Atlanta, United States, the former medical director of the Health Services, Division for Intellectual and Developmental Disabilities, Ministry of Social Affairs and Social Services, Jerusalem, the founder and director of the National Institute of Child Health and Human Development in Israel. Numerous publications in the field of pediatrics, child health and human development, rehabilitation, intellectual disability, disability, health, welfare, abuse, advocacy, quality of life and prevention. Received the Peter Sabroe Child Award for outstanding work on behalf of Danish Children in 1985 and the International LEGO-Prize ("The Children's Nobel Prize") for an extraordinary contribution towards improvement in child welfare and well-being in 1987. Email: jmerrick@zahav.net.il

In: Childhood and Adolescence
Editor: Joav Merrick

ISBN: 978-1-53613-574-9

Chapter 15

About the National Institute of Child Health and Human Development in Israel

The National Institute of Child Health and Human Development (NICHD) in Israel was established in 1998 as a virtual institute under the auspices of the Medical Director, Ministry of Social Affairs and Social Services in order to function as the research arm for the Office of the Medical Director. In 1998 the National Council for Child Health and Pediatrics, Ministry of Health and in 1999 the Director General and Deputy Director General of the Ministry of Health endorsed the establishment of the NICHD.

Mission

The mission of a National Institute for Child Health and Human Development in Israel is to provide an academic focal point for the scholarly interdisciplinary study of child life, health, public health, welfare, disability, rehabilitation, intellectual disability and related aspects of human development. This mission includes research, teaching, clinical work, information and public service activities in the field of child health and human development.

Service and academic activities

Over the years many activities became focused in the south of Israel due to collaboration with various professionals at the Faculty of Health Sciences (FOHS) at the Ben Gurion University of the Negev (BGU). Since 2000 an affiliation with the Zusman Child Development Center at the Pediatric Division of Soroka University Medical Center has resulted in collaboration around the establishment of the Down Syndrome Clinic at that center. In 2002 a full course on "Disability" was established at the Recanati School for Allied Professions in the Community, FOHS, BGU and in 2005 collaboration was started with the Primary Care Unit of the faculty and disability became part of the master of public health course on "Children and society". In the academic year 2005-2006 a one semester course on "Aging with disability" was started as part of the master of science program in gerontology in our collaboration with the Center for Multidisciplinary Research in Aging. In 2010 collaborations with the Division of Pediatrics, Hadassah Hebrew University Medical Center, Jerusalem, Israel around the National Down Syndrome Center and teaching students and residents about intellectual and developmental disabilities as part of their training at this campus.

Research activities

The affiliated staff have over the years published work from projects and research activities in this national and international collaboration. In the year 2000 the International Journal of Adolescent Medicine and Health and in 2005 the International Journal on Disability and Human Development of De Gruyter Publishing House (Berlin and New York) were affiliated with the National Institute of Child Health and Human Development. From

2008 also the International Journal of Child Health and Human Development (Nova Science, New York), the International Journal of Child and Adolescent Health (Nova Science) and the Journal of Pain Management (Nova Science) affiliated and from 2009 the International Public Health Journal (Nova Science) and Journal of Alternative Medicine Research (Nova Science). All peer-reviewed international journals.

National collaborations

Nationally the NICHD works in collaboration with the Faculty of Health Sciences, Ben Gurion University of the Negev; Department of Physical Therapy, Sackler School of Medicine, Tel Aviv University; Autism Center, Assaf HaRofeh Medical Center; National Rett and PKU Centers at Chaim Sheba Medical Center, Tel HaShomer; Department of Physiotherapy, Haifa University; Department of Education, Bar Ilan University, Ramat Gan, Faculty of Social Sciences and Health Sciences; College of Judea and Samaria in Ariel and in 2011 affiliation with Center for Pediatric Chronic Diseases and National Center for Down Syndrome, Department of Pediatrics, Hadassah Hebrew University Medical Center, Mount Scopus Campus, Jerusalem.

International collaborations

Internationally with the Department of Disability and Human Development, College of Applied Health Sciences, University of Illinois at Chicago; Strong Center for Developmental Disabilities, Golisano Children's Hospital at Strong, University of Rochester School of Medicine and Dentistry, New York; Centre on Intellectual Disabilities, University of Albany, New York; Centre for Chronic Disease Prevention and Control, Health Canada, Ottawa; Chandler Medical Center and Children's Hospital, Kentucky Children's Hospital, Section of Adolescent Medicine, University of Kentucky, Lexington; Chronic Disease Prevention and Control Research

Center, Baylor College of Medicine, Houston, Texas; Division of Neuroscience, Department of Psychiatry, Columbia University, New York; Institute for the Study of Disadvantage and Disability, Atlanta; Center for Autism and Related Disorders, Department Psychiatry, Children's Hospital Boston, Boston; Department of Pediatric and Adolescent Medicine, Western Michigan University Homer Stryker MD School of Medicine, Kalamazoo, Michigan, United States; Department of Paediatrics, Child Health and Adolescent Medicine, Children's Hospital at Westmead, Westmead, Australia; International Centre for the Study of Occupational and Mental Health, Düsseldorf, Germany; Centre for Advanced Studies in Nursing, Department of General Practice and Primary Care, University of Aberdeen, Aberdeen, United Kingdom; Quality of Life Research Center, Copenhagen, Denmark; Nordic School of Public Health, Gottenburg, Sweden, Scandinavian Institute of Quality of Working Life, Oslo, Norway; The Department of Applied Social Sciences (APSS) of The Hong Kong Polytechnic University Hong Kong.

Targets

Our focus is on research, international collaborations, clinical work, teaching and policy in health, disability and human development and to establish the NICHD as a permanent institute in Israel in order to conduct model research and provide policy aspects in the field of interest.

Contact

Professor Joav Merrick, MD, MMedSci, DMSc
Former Medical Director, Health Services, Division for Intellectual and Developmental Disabilities, Ministry of Social Affairs and Social Services, POB 1260, IL-91012 Jerusalem, Israel. E-mail: jmerrick@zahav.net.il

In: Childhood and Adolescence
Editor: Joav Merrick
ISBN: 978-1-53613-574-9

Chapter 16

About the Book Series "Pediatrics, Child and Adolescent Health"

Pediatrics, child and adolescent health is a book series with publications from a multidisciplinary group of researchers, practitioners and clinicians for an international professional forum interested in the broad spectrum of pediatric medicine, child health, adolescent health and human development.

- Merrick J, ed. Child and adolescent health yearbook 2011. New York: Nova Science, 2012.
- Merrick J, ed. Child and adolescent health yearbook 2012. New York: Nova Science, 2012.
- Roach RR, Greydanus DE, Patel DR, Homnick DN, Merrick J, eds. Tropical pediatrics: A public health concern of international proportions. New York: Nova Science, 2012.
- Merrick J, ed. Child health and human development yearbook 2011. New York: Nova Science, 2012.
- Merrick J, ed. Child health and human development yearbook 2012. New York: Nova Science, 2012.
- Shek DTL, Sun RCF, Merrick J, eds. Developmental issues in Chinese adolescents. New York: Nova Science, 2012.

- Shek DTL, Sun RCF, Merrick J, eds. Positive youth development: Theory, research and application. New York: Nova Science, 2012.
- Zachor DA, Merrick J, eds. Understanding autism spectrum disorder: Current research aspects. New York: Nova Science, 2012.
- Ma HK, Shek DTL, Merrick J, eds. Positive youth development: A new school curriculum to tackle adolescent developmental issues. New York: Nova Science, 2012.
- Wood D, Reiss JG, Ferris ME, Edwards LR, Merrick J, eds. Transition from pediatric to adult medical care. New York: Nova Science, 2012.
- Isenberg Y. Guidelines for the healthy integration of the ill child in the educational system: Experience from Israel. New York: Nova Science, 2013.
- Shek DTL, Sun RCF, Merrick J, eds. Chinese adolescent development: Economic disadvantages, parents and intrapersonal development. New York: Nova Science, 2013.
- Shek DTL, Sun RCF, Merrick J, eds. University and college students: Health and development issues for the leaders of tomorrow. New York: Nova Science, 2013.
- Shek DTL, Sun RCF, Merrick J, eds. Adolescence and behavior issues in a Chinese context. New York: Nova Science, 2013.
- Sun J, Buys N, Merrick J. Advances in preterm infant research. New York: Nova Science, 2013.
- Tsitsika A, Janikian M, Greydanus DE, Omar HA, Merrick J, eds. Internet addiction: A public health concern in adolescence. New York: Nova Science, 2013.
- Shek, DTL, Lee TY, Merrick J, eds. Promotion of holistic development of young people in Hong Kong. New York: Nova Science, 2013.
- Shek DTL, Ma C, Lu Y, Merrick J, eds. Human developmental research: Experience from research in Hong Kong. New York: Nova Science, 2013.
- Rubin IL, Merrick J, eds. Child health and human development: Social, economic and environmental factors. New York: Nova Science, 2013.

- Merrick J, ed. Chronic disease and disability in childhood. New York: Nova Science, 2013.
- Rubin IL, Merrick J, eds. Break the cycle of environmental health disparities: Maternal and child health aspects. New York: Nova Science, 2013.
- Rubin IL, Merrick J, eds. Environmental health disparities in children: Asthma, obesity and food. New York: Nova Science, 2013.
- Rubin IL, Merrick J, eds. Environmental health: Home, school and community. New York: Nova Science, 2013.
- Merrick J, Kandel I, Omar HA, eds. Children, violence and bullying: International perspectives. New York: Nova Science, 2013.
- Omar HA, Bowling CH, Merrick J, eds. Playing with fire: Children, adolescents and firesetting. New York: Nova Science, 2013.
- Merrick J, Tenenbaum A, Omar HA, eds. School, adolescence and health issues. New York: Nova Science, 2014.
- Merrick J, Tenenbaum A, Omar HA, eds. Adolescence and sexuality: International perspectives. New York: Nova Science, 2014.
- Diamond G, Arbel E. Adoption: The search for a new parenthood adoption. New York: Nova Science, 2014.
- Taylor MF, Pooley JA, Merrick J, eds. Adolescence: Places and spaces. New York: Nova Science, 2014.
- Greydanus DE, Feinberg AN, Merrick J, eds. Born into this world: Health issues. New York: Nova Science, 2014.
- Greydanus DE, Feinberg AN, Merrick J, eds. Caring for the newborn: A comprehensive guide for the clinician. New York: Nova Science, 2014.
- Rubin IL, Merrick J, eds. Environment and hope: Improving health, reducing AIDS and promoting food security in the world. New York: Nova Science, 2014.
- Greydanus DE, Feinberg AN, Merrick J, eds. Pediatric and adolescent dermatology: Some current issues. New York: Nova Science, 2014.

- Roach RR, Greydanus DE, Patel DR, Merrick J, eds. Tropical pediatrics: A public helath concern of international proportions, Second edition. New York: Nova Science, 2015.
- Merrick J, ed. Child and adolescent health issues: A tribute to the pediatrician Donald E Greydanus. New York: Nova Science, 2015.
- Feinberg AN. A pediatric resident pocket guide: Making the most of morning reports. New York: Nova Science, 2015.
- Greydanus DE, Patel DR, Pratt HD, Calles Jr JL, Nazeer A, Merrick J, eds. Behavioral pediatrics, 4th edition. New York: Nova Science, 2015.
- Merrick J, ed. Disability, chronic disease and human development. New York: Nova Science, 2015.
- Hegamin-Younger C, Merrick J, eds. Caribbean adolescents: Some public health concerns. New York: Nova Science, 2015.
- Merrick J, ed. Adolescence and health: Some international perspectives. New York: Nova Science, 2015.
- Omar HA. Youth suicide prevention: Everybody's business. New York: Nova Science, 2015.
- Greydanus DE, Raj VMS, Merrick J, eds. Chronic disease and disability: The pediatric kidney. New York: Nova Science, 2015.
- Merrick J, ed. Children and childhood: Some international aspects. New York: Nova Science, 2016.
- Shek DTL, Lee TY, Merrick J, eds. Children and adolescents: Future challenges. New York: Nova Science, 2016.
- Shek DTL, Wu FKU, Leung JTY, Merrick J, eds. Adolescence: Positive youth development programs in Chinese communities. New York: Nova Science, 2016.
- Merrick J, Greydanus DE, eds. Sexuality: Some international aspects. New York: Nova Science, 2016.
- Harel-Fisch Y, Abdeen Z, Navot M. Growing up in the Middle East: The daily lives and well-being of Israeli and Palestinian youth. New York: Nova Science, 2016.
- Greydanus DE, Malhotra D, Merrick J, eds. Chronic disease and disability: The pediatric heart. New York: Nova Science, 2016.
- Greydanus DE, Kamboj MK, Merrick J, eds. Chronic disease and disability: The pediatric pancreas. New York: Nova Science, 2016.

- Kamboj MK, Greydanus DE, Merrick J, eds. Diabetes mellitus: Childhood and adolescence. New York: Nova Science, 2016.
- Greydanus DE, Palusci VJ, Merrick J, eds. Chronic disease and disability: Abuse and neglect in childhood and adolescence. New York: Nova Science, 2016.
- Greydanus DE, Calles JL Jr, Patel DR, Nazeer A, Merrick J, eds. Clinical aspects of psychopharmacology in childhood and adlescence, second ed. New York: Nova Science, 2016.
- Greydanus DE, Apple RW, White K, Merrick J, eds. Children and youth: Post-traumatic stress disorder and motor vehicle crashes. New York: Nova Science, 2017.
- Mazaba ML, Siziya S, Merrick J, eds. Suicide: A global view on suicidal ideation among adolescents. New York: Nova Science, 2017.
- Chow R, Merrick J, eds. Adolescence: Bicycle and helmet use of adolescents and young adults. New York: Nova Science, 2017.
- Chow R, Borean M, Hollenberg D, Viehweger J, Anpalagan T, Rzepka A, Merrick J, eds. Bicycles: Helmet use and adolescents at independent schools. New York: Nova Science, 2017.
- Shek DTL, Ma CMS, Leung JTY, Merrick J, eds. Positive youth development: Long term effects in a Chinese program. New York: Nova Science, 2017.

Contact

Professor Joav Merrick, MD, MMedSci, DMSc
Medical Director, Medical Services
Division for Intellectual and Developmental Disabilities
Ministry of Social Affairs and Social Services
POBox 1260, IL-91012 Jerusalem, Israel
E-mail: jmerrick@zahav.net.il

SECTION FIVE: INDEX

INDEX

A

academic performance, 20, 67, 116, 118, 121, 123, 124, 125, 127, 129, 131
academic success, 131
activity level, 143, 149, 153, 154, 156, 157, 158, 159, 161
administrative arrangements, 66, 70, 71, 72, 77, 80, 81, 82
adolescent, vii, 4, 5, 6, 11, 12, 20, 21, 22, 23, 27, 29, 31, 48, 51, 57, 58, 62, 66, 67, 68, 74, 83, 84, 92, 93, 94, 95, 98, 99, 100, 102, 104, 105, 106, 108, 109, 110, 111, 112, 113, 114, 115, 118, 128, 129, 132, 133, 134, 135, 215, 228, 229, 231, 232,233, 234
aggression, 21, 142
AIDS, 102, 221, 233
alcohol consumption, 175, 205, 209
alcoholism, 168, 214
America COMPETES Act, 13
anticipatory problem-solving, 116, 117, 121, 130
anxiety, 22, 35, 36, 42, 132, 142, 206, 211, 214
anxiety disorder, 214
APGAR score, 63

B

ban policy, 178, 179, 180, 182, 183, 184, 185
behavioral dispositions, 138
behaviors, 19, 21, 29, 35, 38, 113, 122, 123, 129, 134, 139, 140, 141, 159, 167, 205, 212
belief systems, 164, 165
Birmingham Interview for Maternal Mental Health, 36
birth weight, 48, 51, 52, 55, 56, 58, 62, 63, 202
births, 48, 49, 50, 51, 54, 55, 56, 57, 198
bonding, v, 20, 33, 34, 35, 36, 37, 38, 39, 41, 42, 43, 86, 89
bonding disorder, v, 33, 34, 35, 36, 37, 38, 39, 41
breastfeeding, 39, 188, 197, 198, 200
bullying, 21, 30, 206, 207, 208, 209, 210, 211, 212, 213, 214, 233

C

caesarean section, 37
cancer, 167, 171, 174, 175

child abuse, 34, 162, 205, 207, 210, 211, 212
Child Behavior Checklist, 146
child development, 43, 130
child mortality, 47, 48, 49, 50, 56, 59, 60, 61
child rearing, 35
childhood, 28, 29, 30, 37, 42, 45, 59, 61, 92, 106, 127, 142, 164, 165, 200, 202, 206, 211, 212, 213, 214, 233, 234, 235
Chlamydia trachomatis, 218
chromosomal abnormalities, 52
chronic diseases, 190
cigarette smoking, 175
cognitive development, 200
cognitive impairment, 189
cognitive process, 165
communication, 14, 15, 17, 163, 207, 210
communication patterns, 163
communication skills, 14, 15, 17
comparative analysis, 176
conceptual model, 17
cross-sectional study, 203, 214
cultural influence, 26
culture, 25, 26, 116, 118, 130, 131, 134
curriculum, 17, 26, 71, 76, 80, 232

D

data analysis, 96, 113, 135, 170
data collection, 94, 95, 97, 110, 119, 133
database, 48, 50, 187, 189, 190
delinquent behavior, 21
delinquent friends, 123
demographic characteristics, 98, 134, 161, 190
depression, 37, 39, 43, 44, 132, 139, 141, 142, 163, 165
depressive symptoms, 20
deprivation, 20, 37
developmental disorder, 42
disability, 6, 37, 92, 213, 225, 227, 228, 230, 233, 234, 235
discrimination, 93, 110, 112
diseases, 52, 62, 101, 109, 112, 169, 184, 213, 219
disorder, v, 33, 34, 35, 36, 37, 38, 39, 41, 164, 205, 206, 207, 212, 213, 214, 232, 235
domestic chores, 99
domestic violence, 37, 205, 209, 211, 212
Down syndrome, 6
drug abuse, 40
drug addict, 103

E

EBV infection, 216, 218, 220
education, v, vi, 5, 6, 11, 12, 13, 14, 18, 22, 26, 27, 28, 29, 39, 42, 43, 44, 66, 67, 84, 92, 107, 110, 112, 113, 118, 119, 126, 127, 132, 135, 136, 144, 167, 169, 170, 171, 172, 173, 174, 175, 176, 177, 185, 209, 229
educational policy, 26
educational programs, 169
educational system, 232
educators, 22, 168, 169, 174
Emotional Availability Scales (EAS), 36
emotional health, 16
emotional intelligence, 22, 30
emotional responses, 159
emotionality, 164
empathy, 12, 13, 14, 21, 22, 27, 29, 30
encouragement, 66
enforcement, 178, 180, 183, 184, 185
environment, 16, 67, 94, 107, 109, 140, 185, 207, 209, 210, 211, 212
environmental conditions, 56
environmental factors, 205, 212, 213, 232
Epstein-Barr virus (EBV), 216, 218, 219, 220

exposure, vi, 177, 178, 179, 180, 182, 184, 185, 186
external locus of control, 140, 149, 158
externalizing behavior, 142, 148, 149, 156, 160, 162, 164
extrinsic motivation, 14

F

Facebook, 122, 129
families, 31, 44, 45, 109, 120, 132, 134, 136, 188, 197, 209
family development, 31
family history, 217
family support, 40
family system, 165
fear, 23, 108
feelings, 12, 21, 24, 40, 119, 125
ferritin, 190, 191, 192, 200
fetus, 35, 36
focus group interviews, 118, 120
focus groups, 116, 119, 121, 132, 135

G

gender, vi, 30, 37, 49, 91, 92, 93, 98, 99, 101, 102, 103, 104, 105, 106, 107, 110, 111, 112, 113, 114, 132, 136, 172, 181, 182, 183, 188, 190, 192, 194, 195, 196, 199
gender differences, 99, 101, 113, 132
gender equality, 112
gender identity, 112
gender inequality, 113
gender role, 92, 99, 110, 111
general education, 13
gestation, 48, 50, 52, 58
gestational age, 58, 198
gestures, 208
gifted, 214
giftedness, 212
global health, 62, 178, 188
globalization, 12, 66, 84
good behavior, 23, 25
growth, 34, 52, 94, 107, 163, 189, 199, 200, 202

H

hairy leukoplakia, 216, 218, 221
head and neck cancer, 168, 174, 176
health, v, vi, vii, 3, 4, 5, 6, 7, 9, 16, 27, 29, 31, 33, 35, 37, 39, 40, 41, 42, 43, 44, 45, 47, 48, 49, 56, 57, 58, 60, 61, 62, 66, 67, 83, 84, 85, 91, 92, 93, 95, 96, 98, 101, 102, 103, 104, 105, 106, 107, 108, 110, 111, 112, 113, 114, 133, 134, 135, 160, 162, 167, 168, 169, 170, 172, 173, 174, 175, 176, 177, 178, 179, 184, 185, 187, 188, 189, 190, 194, 196, 197, 199, 200, 201, 206, 212, 213, 214, 215, 220, 221, 225, 227, 228, 229, 230, 231, 232, 233, 234
health care, 61, 62, 103, 104, 108, 110, 199
health education, 5, 6, 135, 172, 175
health information, 104
health problems, 37, 62, 101, 103, 108
health promotion, 5, 168, 169
health services, 4, 5, 93, 103, 188
helicobacter pylori, 188
hematology, 201
hemoglobin, 191
herpes virus, 219
hiatal hernia, 207
high school, 13, 95, 144, 168, 169, 174, 214
high school diploma, 144
higher education, 12, 28, 58
HIV test, 219
HIV/AIDS, 52, 62, 102, 175, 216, 218, 219, 220, 221

human development, 47, 48, 225, 227, 230, 231, 232, 234
human dignity, 24
human experience, 118
human health, 184
human immunodeficiency virus, 216, 221
human immunodeficiency virus (HIV), 52, 62, 102, 175, 216, 218, 219, 220, 221
human interactions, 26, 27
human subjects, 179
hyperactivity, 142, 164, 207, 211, 212
hyperplasia, 218
hypoxia, 52
hysterectomy, 208

I

Ibokun, vi, 177, 178, 179, 180, 184, 185, 186
incubator, 118
infancy, 42, 142, 201, 202
infant feeding practices, 197
infant mortality, 47, 49, 57, 60, 62, 63
infants, vi, 38, 40, 41, 42, 43, 44, 45, 47, 53, 56, 57, 62, 63, 139, 162, 187, 188, 189, 190, 191, 192, 193, 194, 195, 196, 197, 198, 199, 200, 201, 202, 203
infection, 188, 216, 218, 219, 221
instructor quality, 66, 70, 72, 80, 81, 82
internal consistency, 72, 144, 145, 146
internalizing, 142, 148, 149, 156, 160, 162, 164
interpersonal communications, 67
interpersonal relations, 19, 123
interpersonal skills, 16, 17
intervention, v, 33, 34, 37, 38, 39, 40, 41, 42, 43, 44, 103, 158, 172, 202
intervention for bonding disorder, 33, 41
interventional, 168, 169
intrinsic motivation, 14
intrusive parenting, 117
iron, vi, 187, 188, 189, 190, 191, 192, 193, 194, 195, 196, 198, 199, 200, 201, 202, 203

J

Jews, 194, 197

K

kindergarten, 125, 127
Kumar, 35, 42, 43, 63

L

language acquisition, 127
lawnmower parenting, 117
learning, 5, 14, 24, 25, 68, 69, 83, 127, 128, 131, 163, 173
leukoplakia, 218, 220
level of education, 144
lichen planus, 218, 219
Likert scale, 36, 145
literacy, 13
liver function tests, 216, 218
local anesthesia, 208
locus, 140, 145, 148, 149, 151, 153, 154, 156, 157, 158, 159, 161, 164, 165
longitudinal study, 22, 135

M

maltreatment, 211, 214
management, 14, 15, 16, 17, 28, 42, 128
MANOVA, 72, 81
maternal mood, 43, 164
maternal sensitivity, 33, 39, 40, 41, 44, 45
medication, 217, 219
medicine, 4, 6, 220, 231
memory, 140, 210

mental disorder, 35, 39
mental health, 33, 37, 38, 39, 40, 41, 42, 43, 45, 66, 67, 84, 101, 103, 105
Ministry of Education, 42, 67, 84
moral behavior, 23, 24, 26
moral development, 23, 24, 26, 30, 31
moral judgment, 24
moral reasoning, 23, 24
moral standards, 25
morality, 21, 23, 25, 26
mortality, 47, 48, 49, 50, 51, 52, 53, 54, 55, 56, 57, 58, 59, 60, 61, 62, 63
mortality rate, 48, 50, 51, 52, 56, 59, 61
mother-baby relationship, 35, 37
mother-child deprivation, 37
mother-child play, 36
mother-infant bonding disorders, 42
mother-infant bonding questionnaire (MIBQ), 36
mother-infant relationships, 34, 36, 40, 41, 42
Mother-to-Infant Bonding Scale (MIBS), 36
multiple regression analyses, 80, 82, 143
music, 125, 127

N

nervous system, 208
NHS, 215
NIES, 66, 67, 84
nursery school, 163

O

oral hairy leukoplakia (OHL), vi, 215, 216, 217, 218, 219, 220
overparenting, vi, 115, 116, 117, 118, 120, 121, 122, 125, 126, 130, 131, 132, 133, 134, 135
overscheduling, 116, 117, 121, 127

P

P.A.T.H.S., v, 65, 66, 67, 68, 69, 70, 71, 74, 81, 83, 84, 85, 86, 87, 88, 89, 135
parental control, 29, 117, 118, 135, 136
parental demandingness, 117
parental influence, 135
parental responsiveness, 117
parent-child communication, 132, 134
parent-child relationship, 134, 160
parenting, vi, 29, 40, 44, 115, 116, 117, 118, 124, 127, 130, 131, 132, 134, 135, 136, 137, 138, 139, 140, 141, 142, 143, 145, 148, 149, 150, 151, 153, 154, 156, 157, 158, 159, 160, 161, 163, 164
parenting styles, 117, 135, 136
parents, vi, 12, 20, 22, 29, 34, 38, 40, 41, 43, 45, 63, 66, 93, 97, 103, 107, 108, 110, 115, 116, 117, 118, 119, 120, 121, 122, 123, 124, 125, 126, 127, 128, 129, 130, 131, 132, 133, 134, 139, 140, 141, 145, 146, 147, 148, 156, 157, 158, 159, 160, 161, 190, 207,211, 232
participants, 66, 68, 69, 70, 73, 74, 75, 76, 77, 78, 80, 81, 82, 83, 87, 89, 91, 95, 98, 99, 101, 102, 103, 104, 105, 107, 108, 110, 111, 118, 119, 120, 143, 147, 158, 170, 179, 180, 190
pattern coding, 120
peer group, 29
peer relationship, 20, 22, 29, 207
perceived control, 145
perceived self-performance, 66, 72, 81
perinatal, v, 33, 34, 40, 41, 51, 53, 56
personal achievements, 118
personal development, 123, 127
personality, 17, 24, 29, 37, 92, 140, 162, 165
personality characteristics, 92, 165
personality traits, 24, 140
physical abuse, 207, 211, 212

pilot study, vi, 43, 68, 132, 176, 177, 179, 184, 185
PKU, 229
policy, 28, 43, 49, 61, 69, 85, 134, 178, 179, 180, 182, 183, 184, 185, 202, 230
policy responses, 49
positive youth development, 14, 22, 24, 27, 31, 67, 74, 81, 83, 84, 85
postpartum maternal attachment scale, 36
posttraumatic stress, 213
pregnancy, 35, 37, 38, 50, 54, 57, 102, 108, 197
premature death, 61
premature infant, 43, 198
preschool, 147, 165, 200, 210
preschool children, 200
preschoolers, 162, 164
presentation skills, 16
preterm delivery, 58
preterm infants, 38, 50
prevalence rate, 188, 195, 198
prevention, 45, 62, 67, 168, 169, 173, 175, 199, 200, 202, 213, 225, 234
primary school, 126, 128
Project STEEP (Steps Toward Effective and Enjoyable Parenting), 40
prosocial behavior, 20, 21, 29, 30
psychiatry, 34, 84
psychological distress, 43
psychological well-being, 20, 135
psychology, 31, 136, 162
psychometric properties, 146
psychopathology, 165
psychopharmacology, 235
psychosocial competences, 67
psychosomatic, 22
psychotherapy, 39, 40, 41, 43, 44, 45
puberty, 93, 108
public health, 111, 190, 201, 225, 227, 228, 231, 232, 234
public policy, 31, 43

Q

qualitative research, 94, 96, 113, 118, 135
qualitative research approach, 94, 118
quality of life, 189, 225
quality of service, 82
quantitative research, 94
questionnaire, 36, 42, 66, 71, 144, 145, 146, 168, 170, 178, 180, 184

R

reflective function, 33, 39, 40, 41, 44, 138, 161
reflective learning, 68
regression, 79, 138, 151, 152, 155, 156, 157, 160, 162
regression analysis, 156
regression equation, 151, 156, 157
relationship satisfaction, 163
relatives, 207, 209, 211
respiratory distress syndrome, 52, 57, 62
risk, 20, 29, 36, 40, 44, 48, 57, 63, 92, 102, 108, 109, 112, 117, 139, 164, 168, 170, 171, 173, 174, 175, 184, 188, 198, 201, 202, 206, 209, 212, 213, 221
risk factors, 92, 112, 168, 170, 171, 173, 174, 201
rug rat race, 130

S

school, vi, 3, 5, 6, 13, 20, 22, 29, 31, 66, 67, 68, 70, 71, 72, 73, 81, 86, 87, 88, 89, 92, 95, 98, 99, 100, 101, 102, 107, 111, 112, 113, 122, 123, 124, 125, 126, 127, 128, 129, 131, 135, 136, 137, 144, 146, 163, 165, 168, 169, 170, 171, 174, 175, 177, 178, 179, 180, 181, 182, 183, 184, 185,

186, 208, 209, 211, 213, 214, 215, 225, 228, 229, 232, 233, 235
school authority, 169, 170
school performance, 22
school psychology, 113
school success, 131, 135, 136
schooling, 99, 101, 107, 131
secondary education, 119
secondary school students, vi, 122, 168, 175, 177, 179, 184, 185, 186
secondary schools, 68, 70, 71, 81, 107, 122, 127, 175, 178, 179, 180, 185
secondary students, 67
secondhand, vi, 177, 178, 179, 180, 184, 185, 186
self-concept, 145
self-confidence, 15
self-control, 24
self-efficacy, 39, 43
self-esteem, 17, 20
self-identity, 20, 118
self-management, 15, 16, 17, 128
self-reflection, 25, 72, 75, 87, 89
self-regulation, 24, 139
self-reports, 161
self-understanding, 20
sensitivity, 21, 25, 33, 36, 39, 40, 41, 44, 45
SES, 188, 189, 197, 198
sex, 5, 59, 67, 108, 114, 168, 217
sexual activity, 20
sexual behavior, 20, 175
sexual health, 220
sexual intercourse, 216
sexual violence, 108
sexuality, 6, 112, 233
sexually transmitted diseases, 221
sexually transmitted infections, 216, 221
sexually transmitted infections (STIs), 102, 216, 217, 219, 221
smoke, vi, 102, 175, 177, 178, 179, 180, 182, 184, 185, 186
smoke exposure, 175, 179, 184
smoking, 175, 178, 179, 182, 183, 184, 185, 186, 217
social anxiety, 212, 214
social behavior, 19, 21, 164, 165
social behaviour, 92
social circle, 122
social competence, 29
social contract, 23
social desirability, 83
social environment, 209, 210
social exclusion, 112, 114
social interaction, 211
social interactions, 211
social justice, 24
social life, 92, 98, 104, 106, 109, 123
social norms, 23
social psychology, 29, 30
social reality, 118
social relations, 19, 29
social relationships, 19, 29
social responsibility, 13, 14
social skills, 16, 210
social support, 33, 38, 43
socialization, 26, 92, 131, 136, 164
society, 14, 22, 23, 25, 26, 56, 92, 109, 110, 228
socioeconomic status, 158, 188, 201
squamous cell carcinoma, 218, 219
steroids, 217, 219, 220
stress, vi, 41, 109, 137, 138, 139, 141, 142, 143, 145, 148, 149, 150, 151, 153, 154, 156, 157, 158, 159, 160, 161, 162, 164, 207, 211, 235
students, vi, 13, 14, 18, 20, 23, 26, 28, 29, 66, 67, 68, 84, 101, 107, 122, 125, 126, 127, 135, 136, 147, 168, 170, 171, 175, 177, 178, 179, 180, 184, 185, 186, 209, 228, 232
style, 115, 116, 130, 131, 135, 147, 149, 156, 160